AF588147

Cancer Health Disparities

This series of volumes focuses on the complex landscape of cancer health disparities, exploring the multilevel factors contributing to unequal cancer risk and outcomes. Edited and authored by leading experts in the field, volumes provide a rigorous examination of the biological, socioeconomic, behavioral, and systemic determinants that shape the unequal burden of cancer across diverse populations. This series aims to cover current research on and approaches to addressing cancer health disparities, paving the way towards equity in cancer outcomes.

Rodney C. Haring
Editor

Indigenous Genetics, Biobanking, Chemistry, and Cancer Research

Data Talks

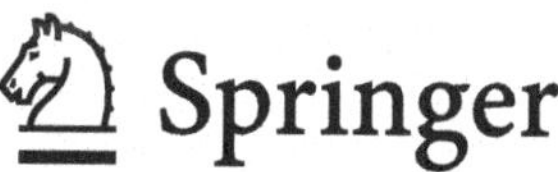

Editor
Rodney C. Haring
Department of Indigenous Cancer Health
Roswell Park Comprehensive Cancer Institute
Buffalo, NY, USA

ISSN 3005-0863 ISSN 3005-0871 (electronic)
Cancer Health Disparities
ISBN 978-3-032-17295-2 ISBN 978-3-032-17296-9 (eBook)
https://doi.org/10.1007/978-3-032-17296-9

This Springer imprint is published by the registered company Springer Nature Switzerland AG
The registered company address is: Gewerbestrasse 11, 6330 Cham, Switzerland

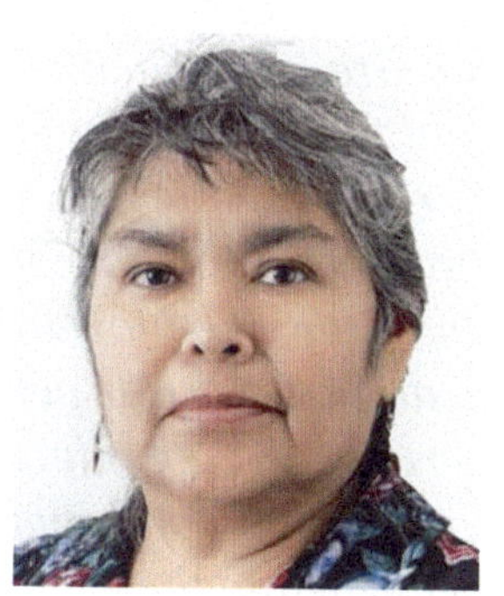

Dr. Francine Gachupin (Pueblo of Jemez, NM), the University of Arizona Cancer Center principal investigator, passed away on September 23, 2024, from stage 4 neuroendocrine carcinoma. Dr. Gachupin had an amazing career as a researcher, mentor, and teacher. She received a Master of Arts degree in Anthropology from the University of New Mexico, a master's in Public Health from the University of Washington, and a doctorate in Anthropology from the University of New Mexico. Dr. Gachupin was a prominent researcher in the field of chronic disease epidemiology and a noted expert in the protection of human research participants, specific to American

Indian biospecimen use in research. She served as founding director of Tribal Epidemiology Centers, chaired several institutional review boards (IRBs), and was committed to education and research founded on the unique needs and strengths of Indigenous communities. Her interdisciplinary work was reflected in her many appointments at the University of Arizona, including Family and Community Medicine, Psychology, American Indian Studies, Public Health, and as a member of the Graduate Faculty. There is so much to be said for Dr. Gachupin's leadership with the Partnership for Native American Cancer Prevention (NACP) and her years of service and dedication toward Native American health equity. Her perseverance will certainly be a guiding light for NACP faculty, staff, and students. This book is dedicated to the memory of our leader, colleague, mentor, and friend, Dr. Francine Gachupin. May she rest in peace.

Foreword

"Ka Ua Hānai Liko"—The Liko Nourishing Rain

The liko (new growth) is nourished by the rain. The rain is much like the knowledge of our ancestors because for us, the liko, to grow, we need the help of the generations that have come before us. A lot of times we separate science and data from Indigenous Knowledge when in actuality, they are one in the same. The knowledge of our ancestors rains down on us and supports our growth. It is also our kuleana (responsibility and privilege) as the new generations to protect and care for the rain, the knowledge, and our kuleana to absorb it and grow stronger than before. To take what has been passed down and turn it into a healthier and stronger tree for the generations to come.

Maliatoa Taualii

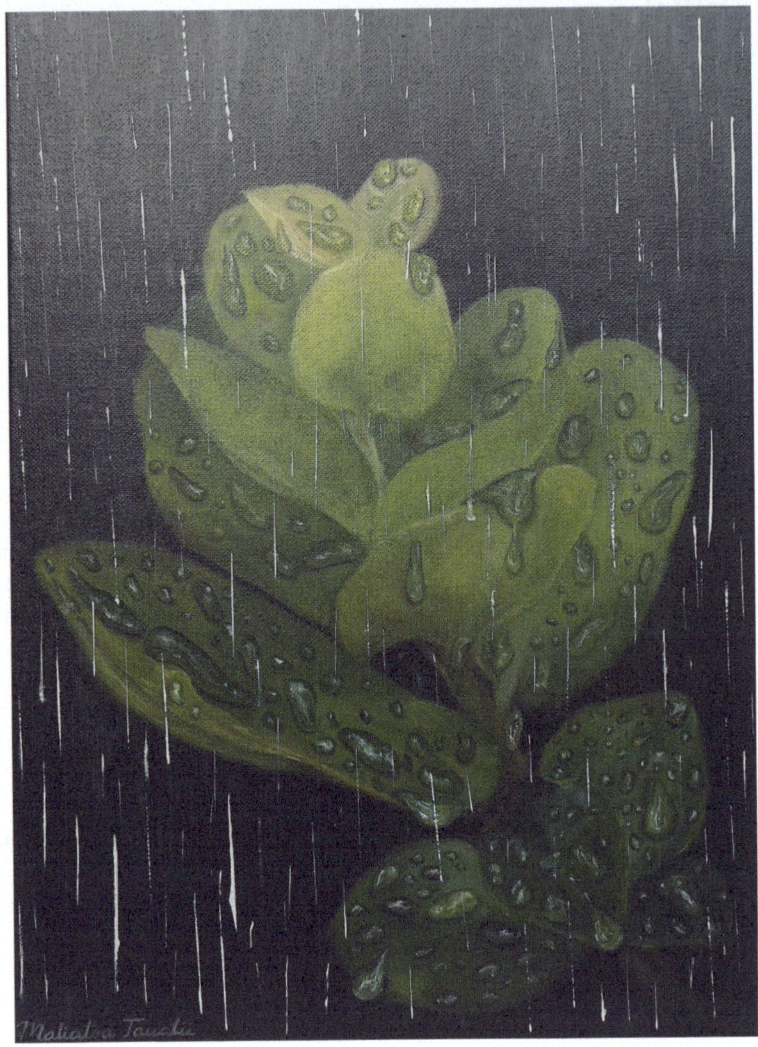

Maliatoa Taualii (Kānaka Maoli) is an artist from Waimānalo on the island of O'ahu. She works with several types of mediums from large-scale murals to wearable art. Her inspiration comes from the desire to move people, to see a new perspective, and to transform them. Much of her art has multiple meanings. In Hawaiian, the word kaona means the deeper meanings and interpretations of something. As such she encourages people to not only look on the surface but also recognize the multiple layers and search for something that resonates with them. She also shares that art is how stories are told and a means to keep Indigenous Knowledge and culture alive.

Preface

Songs of Transparency

The Haudenosaunee (historically known as the Iroquois) tell a story of Creation that explains how SkyWoman fell from the Celestial World onto the back of a Turtle. From there, all life on the Turtle Island (Earth) arose, including people. Yet, from time to time, the Creator visits Turtle Island to see how the world has developed and if the Ongweh'onweh (ongk-way-HON-way), the "real people," are following the instructions we received at the time of Creation. To see if people are using the Good Mind. The relationships between people, nature, the Earth, and the Celestial world is multidirectional and an important part of Haudenosaunee worldview.

Many of the beliefs about these relationships are expressed in the stories the Haudenosaunee have told for generations. One particular story reminds people of the importance of honesty, fair competition, and transparency of behavior.

Long ago, when the Turtle Island was new, the Creator was walking through the forest listening in enjoyment to what had been made. The rustling of leaves as the winds blew created "tree songs," each caressed and supported by the gentle breeze. The water flowed in the streams and created "water songs." In the distance, the Creator heard the Ongweh'onweh singing Thanksgiving songs, the People of the Longhouse giving thanks for everything in the world around them. The Creator smiled as he walked about.

However, as the Creator looked into the sky, he noticed the birds flying in silence but straining to hear the songs around them. They had no songs, no melodies. The Creator called a meeting with the bird leaders, asking if they wanted songs so they could sing Thanksgivings also. The birds were truly excited and affirmed their interest. The Creator agreed to give songs to the birds and told them to assemble the next day. The birds rejoiced with love and appreciation. The Creator smiled.

The following day all the birds assembled. The Creator said there would be great competition. The rules were simple. Whoever flew the highest would be honored with the first song selection. The next highest flyer would get second choice and so on sequentially. The birds agreed and readied themselves for the challenge. As another beautiful sunrise neared, each bird family put forward their greatest aviator. There were the large birds, including the turkey buzzards, hawks, crows, and eagles. The medium-sized birds included robins, jays, and ducks while the smallest birds included sparrows and hummingbirds.

As the morning horizon brightened, the birds excitedly awaited the great flight. Near a stand of tall great white pines, the eagle prepared for the competition. He bragged and boasted about the strength of his wings and the heights he could fly. The other birds, hearing these harsh words, began to worry and wonder if they could compete with the Eagle. One small bird, known as Thrush, worried most of all, knowing his wings were no match for the powerful Eagle. As he prepared, Eagle lay down, rustled his feathers, stretched out his wings, and closed his eyes, deep in thought, reflection, and solitude. Thrush, seeing his opportunity, sneakily hopped onto Eagle's back and nestled himself into a pocket of feathers; he was so small, Eagle never noticed.

The Sun rose above the horizon and the signal to begin was given by the Creator. The birds began to fly!! They soared into the sky in great masses, straining their wings to reach heights they never dreamed they could reach. Soon, the birds began to fall back to Earth. The first to descend was the hummingbird. Others followed but everyone cheered in excitement as each bird had given their best effort. As expected, the Eagle pierced the clouds and had flown the highest. Above the turbulence of the wind, Eagle basked in the serenity of the sky and rejoiced that he had honored the Eagle community. He spiraled down toward the Earth, eager to choose the best song for his family.

But someone else felt this shift in flight as well. Thrush immediately darted out of his hiding place and flew toward the Sun. Eagle was surprised to see someone else so high but had no strength to chase after his rival. He returned to his stand of Great White Pines and informed the other birds, and the Creator, about what Thrush had done. The Creator frowned.

Thrush flew as high as he dared and then excitedly returned to the Earth, ready to select the best song. But as he neared the land, his concern and worry returned. He began to hear jeers and words of dissent, dissatisfaction, and anger. As Thrush landed, the collected birds shared their perspectives of cheating and unfairness. They told Thrush that if he had followed the rules, they would have cheered him but now did not want to hear his song.

The birds gathered to receive their songs. However, the Creator honored his word by granting the Thrush first choice. The eagle selected second and the hummingbird was the last to select a song. To this day, we rejoice to hear Eagle's powerful song honoring truth, strength, protection, and oversight. We also enjoy the quiet wings of hummingbirds in flight, their beautiful "song." But because of his cheating, lack of transparency, and greed to get the best song without respect for others, Thrush rarely shows self. Ashamed, he lives in dark places and is now called Hermit Thrush. On the rare occasion when he does emerge, early in the morning at dawn or toward evening at dusk, Hermit Thrush sings his beautiful song in solitude. When the Haudenosaunee hear him sing, we are reminded of the lesson of how Thrush got such a beautiful song.

This story is a reminder to all people, scientists, and data/wisdom holders that it is important to be honest and transparent in what we do. From a scientific and academic perspective, getting hard to obtain or protected data should not be achieved by cheating, lack of transparency, or thinking with a clouded mind. Rather, it is crucially important to be respectfully curious and/or competitive with a Good Mind—honoring Indigenous Knowledge, truthfulness, and with transparent approaches. This Haudenosaunee teaching translates to modern day practices of academia, health research, grant writing, and data sciences. All too often academics, researchers, universities, cancer centers, and data collection teams are taught Western world practices of competitiveness and competition, pitting institutions against another. Data should not be collected or portrayed only to win a grant. Rather, that data has a story to tell. That story has a collective strength and, with Good Minded intentions, can share lessons and knowledge for generations to come.

The story of how the birds got their songs is a reminder, based in Indigenous Knowledge, that we must be fully transparent in our intentions on how data will be used, how it will be protected, and how data will benefit future generations.

Rochester, NY, USA
Buffalo, NY, USA

Perry Ground
Rodney C. Haring

Acknowledgments

Cancer centers and cancer care organizations across the world serve both dense urban centers and remote rural areas including Indigenous populations. The objective of this book is to advance knowledge in cancer data discussions for and with Indigenous populations and academics, researchers, Nations, institutions, and allies that work with Indigenous cancer data. Chapters will include conversations on current prevalence, incidence, and mortality patterns across populations with overall goals of understanding and utilizing data toward cancer control. Authors will engage in narratives on data as it relates to sovereignty, Indigenous Nation to country to academic institutions with accompanying sections related to citizenship as political classifications along with race, ethnicity, genetics, chemistry, vaccines, cancer data protections, cancer surgery data, small population research methods, and health documentary methods of dissemination. Co-authors, as international leaders in cancer research and allied fields, initiated writings across scientific and community partners from across the world. Combined these processes focused on existing, future, and areas in need of development related to community-based data, Indigenous Knowledge, and cancer control for and with Indigenous communities. "Data Talks" chapters were led by Indigenous scientists, physicians, community members, and health professionals from around the world and form basis for ongoing discussion among scientific data leaders and community-based engagements with key areas including scientific conversations of the state of cancer data science. The overarching goal is to improve the standardization, availability of methods and tools for analysis, protection of data, data ethics, and creation of community-based dissemination processes to build greater understandings of cancer control opportunities based in Indigenous Knowledges and for global Indigenous communities.

This book notates Indigenous populations as American Indian and Alaska Native—AI/AN, Canada (First Nations, Metis, and Inuit), Native Hawaiian and Pacific Islanders with reference to Indigenous Nations, globally. Hence, the word Indigenous will be used throughout the book to represent the many Indigenous or Native Nations across the world. Distinction is woven throughout chapters to honor specific Native Nations and their citizens.

Writings, sharing, and perspectives in this book reflect the international clauses of Springer Publications, Springer Nature, as set forth by their publishing guidelines as situated in the Country of Switzerland. Diversity, equity, and inclusion (DEI) are at the forefront of strategic priorities at Springer Nature and are committed to serving a diverse and global research community. Springer Nature also believes a truly inclusive publishing landscape should represent all communities, globally and across multiple dimensions of diversity. Springer Nature is committed to addressing gender imbalance in research and publishing (Retrieved, August 8, 2025, from https://www.springernature.com/gp/editors/resources-tools/dei-for-editors).

Research, writing, quality improvement, and perspectives shared in this publication were supported by numerous federal, private, and philanthropic funding sources and are solely the responsibilities of the authors. They do not represent the official views of any federal health system, cancer center, university, or government. For more information, reference, and citation of grant support, please reach out to respective chapter authors.

Contents

About the Editors

Rodney C. Haring, PhD, MSW (Seneca, Beaver Clan) is inaugural Chair of the Department of Indigenous Cancer Health at Roswell Park Comprehensive Cancer Center. He is an enrolled member of the Seneca Nation of Indians and resides on the Cattaraugus Indian Reservation (NY). He holds a doctoral degree in social work with over 15 years of social work practice and a former delegate on the US Department of Health and Human Services, American Indian and Alaska Native, Health Research Advisory Council. He is also the lead delegate for the historic MoU between Rowell Park and Indian Health Services with the common mission of addressing health burdens in Indigenous communities. In 2017, he was awarded an Impact Award by the National Indian Health Board, and in 2021, he received the National Federation of Just Communities Hero Award. His research interests intersect eliminating disparities and encouraging resiliencies within First Nations and Indigenous societies.

Community Engagement to Improve Cancer Outcomes Among American Indian and Alaska Native Communities

Jessica W. Blanchard, Paul G. Spicer, Bobby Saunkeah, Lancer D. Stephens, Evelyn D. Cox, Kristen Wilson, Mark P. Doescher, Dorothy A. Rhoades, and Vanessa Y. Hiratsuka

Abstract Many American Indian and Alaska Native (AI/AN) Tribes and their citizens view health research as an important component in their strategies to address well-known and widely documented health disparities. AI/AN community interest in improving health through participation in research carries an important caveat—that continuous, meaningful, and transparent community engagement also occur. AI/AN community involvement in the initiation of research, AI/AN community member participation in manuscript development, and the use of AI/AN regulatory agreements in the conduct of research are key features from participatory research that are frequently absent, undercutting respect for the sovereign authority of Tribal Nations to govern research in their communities (e.g., ensure the protection and oversight of their data in the research process). A community-engaged approach to cancer research requires time, trust, teamwork, and resources that are not always

J. W. Blanchard (✉)
Center for Applied Social Research, University of Oklahoma, Norman, OK, USA
e-mail: jessicawalker@ou.edu

P. G. Spicer
Department of Anthropology, University of Oklahoma, Norman, OK, USA
e-mail: paul.spicer@ou.edu

B. Saunkeah
Division of Research, Chickasaw Nation Department of Health, Ada, OK, USA
e-mail: Bobby.Saunkeah@chickasaw.net

L. D. Stephens
Hudson College of Public Health, University of Oklahoma Health Campus, Oklahoma City, OK, USA
e-mail: lancer-stephens@ouhsc.edu

E. D. Cox
Native Nations Center for Tribal Policy Research, School of Library and Information Studies, University of Oklahoma, Norman, OK, USA
e-mail: ecox@ou.edu

R. C. Haring (ed.), *Indigenous Genetics, Biobanking, Chemistry, and Cancer Research*, Cancer Health Disparities, https://doi.org/10.1007/978-3-032-17296-9_1

supported by research institutions; in fact, many institutional procedures for research can create barriers to the time, trust, and commitment needed for community-engaged research with Tribal populations. In this chapter, the authors describe community engagement efforts within the University of Oklahoma Stephenson Cancer Center's initiative to Improve Cancer Outcomes in Native American Communities (ICON).

Keywords Community engagement · Cancer research · American Indian/Alaska Native · Community–institutional relations · Community participation

Abbreviations

AI/AN	American Indian/Alaska Native
CEIGR	Center for the Ethics of Indigenous Genomic Research
COE	Community Outreach and Engagement
ICON	Improve Cancer Outcomes in Native American Communities
NACCHE	Native American Center for Cancer Health Excellence
OCTSI	Oklahoma Clinical and Translational Sciences Institute
SCC	Stephenson Cancer Center

Many American Indian and Alaska Native (AI/AN) Tribes and their citizens view health research as an important component in their strategies to address well-known and widely documented health disparities (Davis & Reid, 1999; Redvers et al., 2024). This interest in improving health through participation in research carries an

K. Wilson
Native American Center for Cancer Health Excellence, Stephenson Cancer Center, University of Oklahoma Health Campus, Oklahoma City, OK, USA
e-mail: Kristen-Wilson-1@ouhsc.edu

M. P. Doescher
Department of Family and Preventive Medicine, Stephenson Cancer Center, University of Oklahoma Health Campus, Oklahoma City, OK, USA
e-mail: Mark-Doescher@ouhsc.edu

D. A. Rhoades
Department of Internal Medicine, Native American Center for Cancer Health Excellence, University of Oklahoma Health Campus, Oklahoma City, OK, USA
e-mail: Dorothy-Rhoades@ouhsc.edu

V. Y. Hiratsuka
Research Department, Southcentral Foundation, Anchorage, AK, USA
e-mail: vhiratsuka@southcentralfoundation.com

important caveat—that continuous, meaningful, and transparent community engagement also occur (Mainous 3rd et al., 2023; Mello & Wolf, 2010; Pacheco et al., 2013). Continuous engagement is not the same as continuous presence. Engagement should be dedicated to community preferences, be articulated through AI/AN governance, and be part of a thoughtful strategy for how engagement will contribute to community-defined positive outcomes and impacts (Hearod et al., 2019).

A 2024 scoping review of AI/AN randomized clinical trials research found that quality community engagement with AI/AN people includes early community involvement in study design, implementation of culturally tailored recruitment strategies, and dissemination of research findings in formats accessible to AI/AN communities (Redvers et al., 2024). Another scoping review found that key aspects of community engagement were frequently absent in participatory research with AI/AN communities, including AI/AN community involvement in the initiation of research, AI/AN community member participation in manuscript development, and the use of AI/AN regulatory agreements in the conduct of research (Woodbury et al., 2019b).

The absence of these key features from participatory research with AI/AN communities also undercuts respect for the sovereign authority of Tribal Nations to govern research in their communities and to ensure the protection and oversight of their data in the research process. The unique political status of AI/AN Nations is rooted in an inherent sovereignty, i.e., at a minimum, a legal construct, a political designation, and a cultural framework whereby "Native people articulate the affirmative content of their inherent sovereignty" through lived experience and practice (Tsosie, 2002). Tribal sovereignty is upheld in courts but, perhaps increasingly vital for community-engaged research, sovereignty is also conferred through value-based, community-grounded practices that provide pathways to sustain and empower communities and ensure that the conduct of research is guided by connections that matter in everyday practice (Harjo, 2019). Authentic community engagement in Tribal contexts insists on outside researchers having continuing education about and respect for sovereignty in research.

As Chadwick et al. note, "as sovereign nations, Tribes have the unquestioned legal right and authority to govern their people, including the right to approve and monitor research conducted within their nations" (Chadwick et al., 2019). This collective responsibility, which is a reflection of Tribes' historical struggles for survival, provides the moral legitimacy to their efforts to protect the whole Tribe by controlling research activities conducted in their communities (Saunkeah et al., 2021). The justice principle of solidarity obligates tribes to fulfill their ethical duties to promote and protect community interests (Saunkeah et al., 2021). The regulation of research by Tribes includes exercising self-determination via the development of Tribal research codes, Tribal Institutional Review Boards, and Tribal research departments (Garba et al., 2023), but equally important are the efforts of researchers at non-Tribal research institutions to conduct themselves in a manner that is respectful of Tribes and Tribal values. Research conducted by researchers at non-Tribal institutions, especially those with no experience or active relationships with Tribal partners, requires the development and maintenance of trusting and equitable relationships in which to understand and apply respectful practices (Blanchard & Hiratsuka, 2021).

Respect is "mutually empowering" and demonstrates a consideration of the ideas of Tribal partners (Tsosie et al., 2024). Past federal initiatives underscore the importance of respect for Indigenous ways of knowing (House, 2022). This is a welcome and necessary direction for cancer research in AI/AN communities, especially considering persistent hesitations by some AI/AN peoples to participate in basic science research. Research infrastructures that fail to promote authentic community engagement aligned with the values and experiences of communities perpetuate harmful research practices, including the failure to properly consent, the unauthorized sharing of data, community stigmatization, and others (Bowekaty & Davis, 2003; Christopher et al., 2011; Drabiak-Syed, 2010; Harding et al., 2012; Hodge, 2012; Lemke et al., 2022; Morton et al., 2013; Strickland, 2006). In the case of genomic research, for example, some AI/AN communities have expressed willingness to participate if appropriate safeguards are in place, which often involve "protecting community interests and ensuring that communities receive some tangible health benefit from participation," as well as control over primary and secondary uses of biological samples and associated data (Beans et al., 2020; Carroll et al., 2022; Chadwick et al., 2019; Dirks et al., 2019; Garrison & Carroll, 2023; Hudson et al., 2020; Trinidad et al., 2022).

It is more important that evaluation protocols and funding review processes similarly encourage the use of evaluation measures that validate Indigenous values, ways of knowing, and notions of success (Bowman & Bremner, 2025; Lafrance, 2004; Lafrance & Nichols, 2008). Health research with AI/AN communities has often been viewed through the lens of a *deficits model* that reinforces gaps in research programs, slow growth, lack of Tribal capacity, or challenging partnerships that struggle to reach conventional benchmarks (Kennedy et al., 2022). The evaluation and conduct of new and ongoing research with AI/AN communities should instead establish measures defined by community interests and the needs of Tribal partners (Bowman & Bremner, 2025).

Standardized metrics to assess the quality of community engagement have also been absent from many models and processes, leaving partners without indicators and measures to discuss, improve, and sustain engagement (Mrklas et al., 2023). Standardized criteria for evaluating community engagement with AI/AN may not appear standardized at all (Bowman & Bremner, 2025), as is expected when input from institutionally marginalized communities begins to directly shape the research process. Recent years have seen substantial innovation in models of community engagement in health research generally, and with AI/AN communities specifically (Woodbury et al., 2019b). Community engagement, including ongoing investment in forging trustful and equitable relationships, is a conduit for good research and improved health outcomes (Yarborough et al., 2013). The pathways needed to engage communities as partners in research are often the same pathways for improving the prevention, screening, and treatment of cancers (Thomas et al., 2024). A community-engaged approach to cancer research requires time, trust, teamwork, and resources that are not always supported by research institutions; in fact, many institutional procedures for research can create barriers to the time, trust, and commitment needed for community-engaged research with Tribal populations (Blanchard & Hiratsuka, 2021; Blanchard et al., 2015; Gittelsohn et al., 2020; James et al., 2014; Kowalkowski et al., 2022; Lucero et al., 2020; Marrero et al., 2013).

Improve Cancer Outcomes in Native American Communities (ICON) Recently funded by the National Institute for Minority Health and Health Disparities, the Stephenson Cancer Center's initiative to *I*mprove *C*ancer *O*utcomes in *N*ative American Communities (ICON) is a 5-year effort to develop research to address significant sources of cancer disparities in Tribal communities. ICON includes projects to (1) understand environmental risk for cancer, (2) improve access to cancer screening, and (3) increase care coordination between Indian Health Service/Tribal/Urban (ITU) systems and the Stephenson Cancer Center (SCC), an NCI-designated cancer center. This work is united by a focus on improving community engagement with Native Nations.

The goal for ICON is to establish and celebrate the space where AI/AN community-engaged research can flourish, by advancing approaches to community engagement that sustain and grow existing partnerships and create the institutional scaffolding needed to support cancer research that is inclusive of Tribal input and Tribal priorities and fully supportive of Tribal sovereignty. ICON emphasizes engagement that is co-equal, co-created, culturally centered, trust building, inclusive, responsive, multidirectional, and founded on respect for Tribal sovereignty (Saunkeah et al., 2021).

Through multiple years of work in collaboration with Tribal populations, ICON is founded upon a rich environment that has already supported multiple partnerships for health research: the SCC Native American Center for Cancer Health Excellence (NACCHE), SCC Community Outreach and Engagement (COE), the Oklahoma Clinical and Translational Sciences Institute (OCTSI), the OCTSI Tribal Engagement Unit, and the University of Oklahoma Native Nations Center for Tribal Policy Research. The investigators and staff at these academic centers have developed multiple Tribal Nation and community organization collaborations, partnerships, and events that demonstrate an ongoing commitment and investment in building capacity for Tribal outreach and engagement. The University of Oklahoma has also received funding for a national Center of Excellence from the National Human Genome Research Institute specifically to support continued innovation in community engagement in AI/AN communities, the Center for the Ethics of Indigenous Genomic Research (CEIGR).

ICON's efforts are supported by a plan for regularly eliciting, synthesizing, and applying community feedback for continuous improvement in community engagement as work toward the kinds of partnerships that Native communities expect and deserve are pursued. As health research with Tribal Nations has grown, there is also a critical need to address the increasing demands on Tribal community partners.

The core of this approach to community engagement has been articulated in the context of CEIGR, which is a multidisciplinary consortium of community-placed Tribal partners, university researchers, and community-based institutions working collaboratively to conduct ethical, legal, and social implications of research in AI/AN communities in the United States. CEIGR emerged in response to the persistent, unresolved issues that kept many Tribal Nations from participating in genomic research (Blanchard et al., 2020; Hiratsuka et al., 2020b). Recognizing that the decision not to participate may remain the best choice for many communities, it was also understood that failures to authentically engage AI/AN communities and recognize Tribal rights to self-governance may also contribute to barriers that may still be resolved (Burke et al., 2022). This understanding elevated a commitment to pursue engagement in ways that promoted increased representation, dialogue, and inclusion of AI/AN researchers and community perspectives (Hiratsuka et al., 2020c; Woodbury et al., 2019a), resulting in a series of important contributions to the literature on community engagement in Tribal communities, especially in the innovative approach to deliberation that was developed through CEIGR (Beans et al., 2019, 2020; Blacksher et al., 2021; Blanchard et al., 2020; Hiratsuka et al., 2020a, b; Woodbury et al., 2019a, 2020). CEIGR developed innovative approaches to engage diverse perspectives, promote wide-ranging discussion within and between communities, and respect the sovereignty and heterogeneity of AI/AN people. These approaches will continue through ICON's community engagement core activities.

Following principles of engagement as described, ICON's emphasis is on engagement that is co-equal, co-created, culturally centered, trust building, inclusive, responsive, multidirectional, and founded on respect for Tribal sovereignty (Saunkeah et al., 2021). Community engagement strategies will draw on innovative approaches developed in the contexts noted above. Central to these efforts is the continued development of organizational structures to improve engagement with diverse segments of AI/AN communities served by ICON. This includes working with multiple preexisting and new Indigenous community advisory boards and collaborations, as well as Tribal institutional structures in a way that minimizes burden on Tribal community partners and maximizes efficiency.

The goal is to streamline processes for forging connections between the SCC and the communities served. Establishing explicit channels for collaboration enables communities interested in cancer-related research to find trustworthy partners from ICON and for SCC researchers with expertise relevant to community partners to find community connections. Minimally, this effort includes (1) regular assessments of SCC cancer research through SCC/NACCHE's Tribal Advisory Council, (2) ongoing epidemiological surveillance through COE, and (3) work with Tribal partners through the SCC/NACCHE Tribal Advisory Committee to recurrently understand and modify cancer research priorities in Oklahoma. It also includes the embedding of Community Engagement Core faculty and staff on research project teams, especially in their interactions with Community Advisory Boards, to ensure that lessons learned within these established partnerships are channeled into continuous improvement for the broader set of ICON activities. Adjusting these approaches to community engagement based on the impact they have on community partners is a paramount concern in implementing the work of ICON. Facilitating bidirectional communication about cancer outcomes research priorities permits the continued organization of SCC and NACCHE to more effectively respond to the needs of Tribal Nations.

Engagement Studios ICON is focused on creating capacity for investigators interested in partnering with Native communities to engage with them in advance of developing their research. Engagement Studios, modeled on the Community Engagement Studios developed by the Meharry-Vanderbilt Community-Engaged Research Core, provide a structured method for establishing collaboration channels between community partners and research teams to enhance the design, conduct, and dissemination of research (Joosten et al., 2015). All too often researchers seek statements of Tribal support for fully formed projects without prior community input and collaboration (Norström et al., 2020). In many cases, these fully formed projects can be contingently approved by institutional review boards or even funded with only a stated goal that the investigators will seek human subjects approval or engage community partners. Omitting community input and Tribal authority at the most fundamental stages of research design undermines the potential for equity and sovereignty in research.

Engagement studios prioritize multidirectional engagement with community partners to inform the development, implementation, and dissemination of research (Joosten et al., 2015). In the context of cancer research, the structured and facilitated forums of engagement studios create space for valuable insights for enhancing community engagement in health research and clinical trials (Killough et al., 2024). Engagement studios consist of panels of community partners from a geographic region, representing multiple Tribal nations who consult on project design and provide guidance from their Tribal communities and lived experience in their Tribal cultures. Engagement studios panelists are not researchers, or even research participants, but are compensated collaborators whose feedback and direction are instrumental in the development and dissemination of research protocols as they bring a layperson's point of view and concern. Engagement studios allow a collaborative format, deeply seeded in respect for all, and advance dialogue on matters of project design and protocol development, implementation, consideration on special topics, and other emergent issues that may be unknown to researchers. An overarching outcome of the engagement studios is to establish a broader institutional culture of collaboration in cancer research. The benefits of using engagement studios go beyond the goals of just improving a given researcher's project or translating scientific outcomes to diverse community audiences. The engagement studios structure relies on the participation of multiple partner groups—both academic and community groups—and cooperative efforts to reach a shared vision for research, a foundation of mutual trust, cultural humility, and mutual benefit from research (Israel et al., 2018).

Accelerators Following the model articulated based on work at Mt. Sinai (Partners, 2025), ICON organizes groups of academic and community collaborators to address select topics geared toward improvements in public health and health care. Just as engagement studios foster collaboration and multidirectional communication between academic and community partners, they also tend to be reserved for addressing complicated problems of research design that require ample time for co-learning, inclusion of multiple perspectives, and trust building (Joosten et al., 2015). As ICON grows its research portfolio, there will be many occasions to address issues, concerns, and questions that emerge in the context of doing research in dynamic environments, especially related to translation in identified areas of emphasis: cancer prevention, cancer screening, and cancer care coordination. Often these emergent issues need prompt consideration that does not allow for the time and structure needed for engagement studios. Accelerators are designed to offer "flexible, readied catalytic frameworks designed to foster communication across scientific and non-scientific divides…" that promote "timely responsiveness to pressing questions, resulting in the more rapid generation of novel solutions to address and ultimately eliminate disparities" (Horowitz et al., 2017). Accelerators for ICON will involve the same network of partners as is used in engagement studios, but with a goal of working together to spark rapid innovation on specific solutions and emergent topics related to the translation of research into action to improve AI/AN cancer outcomes.

Integration with Navigation and Outreach at NACCHE As described above, the ICON CE Core is embedded in SCC and NACCHE's rich environment for improving AI/AN cancer health excellence, with SCC's American Indian Navigation service (itself a focus of an ICON Project) and NACCHE's team of Tribal Outreach Liaisons. Both workforces are focused on improving AI/AN cancer outcomes, so it is vital for close contact between these services to ensure that identified problems can be responded efficiently. While longer term efforts to improve cancer outcomes will unfold in the context of ICON research, there is likely no shortage of immediate practice improvements that will be generated and can be acted upon quickly in the context of ICON community engagements and Tribal health research settings if those settings have dedicated and sustainable research infrastructure and dedicated research staff (e.g., research coordinators, recruiters, etc.).

Community Forums on SCC Native American Cancer Research One of the consistent failures in community-engaged research in Tribal communities relates to the return of results to communities. Whereas select Tribal partners and community collaborators are identified for repeat participation in the Engagement Studios and the Accelerators, Community Forums present an option for broader participation by community members who may not be participating in other engagement outlets but nonetheless should have the opportunity to learn about and respond to ongoing cancer research initiatives. ICON employs an approach to Community Forums developed by an Alaska Native health organization for sharing Tribally-directed research findings (Hiratsuka et al., 2018a, b), and further adapted with Tribal partners as part of work with CEIGR. Community Forums are single-day events, happening over a 3- to 4-h period, designed to showcase components of research (e.g., oral presentations, lightning talks, distribution of project materials, poster presentations, and other formats) that are then subject to facilitated group discussion with designated periods of community questions and feedback.

ICON's Community Forums provide platforms for multidirectional communication about the research process, presentations from researchers to community, additional expert presenters as needed, discussion among community participants only, and reporting out feedback from community participants to researchers (Hiratsuka et al., 2018b). Forums are carefully designed in consultation with Tribal partners to ensure that they address a defined issue or question and include small and large group activities structured to facilitate robust and truly bidirectional dialogue around those issues (Hiratsuka et al., 2018a). These forums are also designed to inform additional dissemination efforts as well, providing communities with the opportunity to shape future ICON Projects, and recruit additional members of Engagement Studio and Accelerator participation. These will include various communication channels including presentations at local, state, and national community and professional meetings; peer-reviewed publications and lay summaries; dashboards, infographics, and videos; and other strategies identified through discussions with community members in these forums.

ICON has established a team that is in regular conversation regarding expanded community engagement for cancer research at the SCC. The team meets weekly, addresses internal and external challenges, and plans events for ICON. Through multiple years of refining engagement strategies, ICON has succeeded in bringing multiple entities that engage Oklahoma Tribal communities into conversation and has developed a coordinated approach to maintain and grow these relationships without overburdening Tribal community partners. The ultimate goal is to improve the health of Tribal people by addressing cancer prevention, screening, and care coordination.

Acknowledgments The research reported in this publication was supported by the National Institute on Minority Health and Health Disparities of the National Institutes of Health under Award Number U19MD020537. The content is solely the responsibility of the authors and does not necessarily represent the official views of the National Institutes of Health.

References

Beans, J. A., Saunkeah, B., Brian Woodbury, R., Ketchum, T. S., Spicer, P. G., & Hiratsuka, V. Y. (2019). Community protections in American Indian and Alaska native participatory research-a scoping review. *Social Sciences, 8*(4). https://doi.org/10.3390/socsci8040127

Beans, J. A., Woodbury, R. B., Wark, K. A., Hiratsuka, V. Y., & Spicer, P. (2020). Perspectives on precision medicine in a tribally managed primary care setting. *AJOB Empirical Bioethics, 11*(4), 246–256. https://doi.org/10.1080/23294515.2020.1817172

Blacksher, E., Hiratsuka, V. Y., Blanchard, J. W., Lund, J. R., Reedy, J., Beans, J. A., et al. (2021). Deliberations with American Indian and Alaska native people about the ethics of genomics: An adapted model of deliberation used with three tribal communities in the United States. *AJOB Empirical Bioethics, 12*(3), 164–178. https://doi.org/10.1080/23294515.2021.1925775

Blanchard, J., & Hiratsuka, V. (2021). Being in good community: Engagement in support of indigenous sovereignty. *The American Journal of Bioethics, 21*(10), 54–56. https://doi.org/10.1080/15265161.2021.1965243

Blanchard, J. W., Petherick, J. T., & Basara, H. (2015). Stakeholder engagement: A model for tobacco policy planning in Oklahoma tribal communities. *American Journal of Preventive Medicine, 48*(1 Suppl 1), S44–S46. https://doi.org/10.1016/j.amepre.2014.09.025

Blanchard, J., Hiratsuka, V., Beans, J. A., Lund, J., Saunkeah, B., Yracheta, J., et al. (2020). Power sharing, capacity building, and evolving roles in ELSI: The Center for the Ethics of indigenous genomic research. *Collaborations (Coral Gables, Fla.), 3*(1). https://doi.org/10.33596/coll.71

Bowekaty, M. B., & Davis, D. S. (2003). Cultural issues in genetic research with American Indian and Alaskan native people. *IRB: Ethics & Human ResearchIRB, 25*(4), 12–15.

Bowman, N., & Bremner, L. (2025). Indigenous data sovereignty: Applying it by, with, for, and through indigenous evaluators and evaluations. *Canadian Journal of Program Evaluation, 39*. https://doi.org/10.3138/cjpe-2024-0039

Burke, W., Beans, J. A., Cho, M. K., Garrison, N. A., Hiratsuka, V., Hopkins, S., et al. (2022). Values and practices to strengthen genetic research partnerships with indigenous communities. *Progress in Community Health Partnerships: Research, Education, and Action, 16*(4), 583–592. https://doi.org/10.1353/cpr.2022.0079

Carroll, S. R., Garba, I., Plevel, R., Small-Rodriguez, D., Hiratsuka, V. Y., Hudson, M., & Garrison, N. A. (2022). Using indigenous standards to implement the CARE principles: Setting expectations through tribal research codes. *Frontiers in Genetics, 13*, 823309. https://doi.org/10.3389/fgene.2022.823309

Chadwick, J. Q., Copeland, K. C., Branam, D. E., Erb-Alvarez, J. A., Khan, S. I., Peercy, M. T., et al. (2019). Genomic research and American Indian tribal communities in Oklahoma: Learning from past research misconduct and building future trusting partnerships. *American Journal of Epidemiology, 188*(7), 1206–1212. https://doi.org/10.1093/aje/kwz062

Christopher, S., Saha, R., Lachapelle, P., Jennings, D., Colclough, Y., Cooper, C., et al. (2011). Applying indigenous community-based participatory research principles to partnership development in health disparities research. *Family & Community Health, 34*(3), 246–255. https://doi.org/10.1097/FCH.0b013e318219606f

Davis, S. M., & Reid, R. (1999). Practicing participatory research in American Indian communities. *The American Journal of Clinical Nutrition, 69*(4 Suppl), 755s–759s. https://doi.org/10.1093/ajcn/69.4.755S

Dirks, L. G., Shaw, J. L., Hiratsuka, V. Y., Beans, J. A., Kelly, J. J., & Dillard, D. A. (2019). Perspectives on communication and engagement with regard to collecting biospecimens and family health histories for cancer research in a rural Alaska native community. *Journal of Community Genetics, 10*(3), 435–446. https://doi.org/10.1007/s12687-019-00408-9

Drabiak-Syed, K. (2010). *Lessons from Havasupai tribe v. Arizona State University Board of Regents: Recognizing Group, Cultural, and Dignitary Harms as Legitimate Risks Warranting Integration into Research Practice*. Retrieved from WorldCat database.

Garba, I., Sterling, R., Plevel, R., Carson, W., Cordova-Marks, F. M., Cummins, J., et al. (2023). Indigenous peoples and research: Self-determination in research governance. *Frontiers in Resonance Metrology and Analysis, 8*, 1272318. https://doi.org/10.3389/frma.2023.1272318

Garrison, N. A., & Carroll, S. R. (2023). Genetic research with indigenous peoples: Perspectives on governance and oversight in the US. *Frontiers in Research Metrics and Analytics, 8*, 1286948. https://doi.org/10.3389/frma.2023.1286948

Gittelsohn, J., Belcourt, A., Magarati, M., Booth-LaForce, C., Duran, B., Mishra, S. I., et al. (2020). Building capacity for productive indigenous community-university partnerships. *Prevention Science, 21*(Suppl 1), 22–32. https://doi.org/10.1007/s11121-018-0949-7

Harding, A., Harper, B., Stone, D., O'Neill, C., Berger, P., Harris, S., & Donatuto, J. (2012). Conducting research with tribal communities: Sovereignty, ethics, and data-sharing issues. *Environmental Health Perspectives, 120*(1), 6–10. https://doi.org/10.1289/ehp.1103904

Harjo, L. (2019). Spiral to the stars: Mvskoke tools of futurity. In *Critical issues in indigenous studies*. Retrieved from https://www.jstor.org/stable/10.2307/j.ctvh4zjdg

Hearod, J. B., Wetherill, M. S., Salvatore, A. L., & Bird Jernigan, V. B. (2019). Community-based participatory intervention research with American Indian communities: What is the state of the science? *Current Developments in Nutrition, 3*, 39–52. https://doi.org/10.1093/cdn/nzz008

Hiratsuka, V. Y., Avey, J. P., Beans, J. A., Dirks, L. G., Caindec, K., & Dillard, D. A. (2018a). Approach and methods of the 2016 Alaska native research forum. *American Indian and Alaska Native Mental Health Research, 25*(1), 19–29. https://doi.org/10.5820/aian.2501.2018.19

Hiratsuka, V. Y., Beans, J. A., Dirks, L. G., Avey, J. P., Caindec, K., & Dillard, D. A. (2018b). Alaska Native Health Research Forum: Perspectives on disseminating research findings. *American Indian and Alaska Native Mental Health Research, 25*(1), 30–41. https://doi.org/10.5820/aian.2501.2018.30

Hiratsuka, V. Y., Beans, J. A., Blanchard, J. W., Reedy, J., Blacksher, E., Lund, J. R., & Spicer, P. G. (2020a). An Alaska native community's views on genetic research, testing, and return of results: Results from a public deliberation. *PLoS One, 15*(3), e0229540. https://doi.org/10.1371/journal.pone.0229540

Hiratsuka, V. Y., Beans, J. A., Reedy, J., Yracheta, J. M., Peercy, M. T., Saunkeah, B., et al. (2020b). Fostering ethical, legal, and social implications research in tribal communities: The Center for the Ethics of indigenous genomic research. *Journal of Empirical Research on Human Research Ethics, 15*(4), 271–278. https://doi.org/10.1177/1556264619872640

Hiratsuka, V. Y., Hahn, M. J., Woodbury, R. B., Hull, S. C., Wilson, D. R., Bonham, V. L., et al. (2020c). Alaska native genomic research: Perspectives from Alaska native leaders, federal staff, and biomedical researchers. *Genetics in Medicine, 22*(12), 1935–1943. https://doi.org/10.1038/s41436-020-0926-y

Hodge, F. S. (2012). No meaningful apology for American Indian unethical research abuses. *Ethics & Behavior, 22*(6), 431–444. https://doi.org/10.1080/10508422.2012.730788

Horowitz, C. R., Shameer, K., Gabrilove, J., Atreja, A., Shepard, P., Goytia, C. N., et al. (2017). Accelerators: Sparking innovation and transdisciplinary team science in disparities research. *International Journal of Environmental Research and Public Health, 14*(3). https://doi.org/10.3390/ijerph14030225

House, T. W. (2022). *Readout: Engagement on development of white House indigenous knowledge effort*. Retrieved from https://bidenwhitehouse.archives.gov/ostp/news-updates/2022/06/27/readout-ostp-and-ceq-initial-engagement-on-white-house-indigenous-knowledge-effort/

Hudson, M., Garrison, N. A., Sterling, R., Caron, N. R., Fox, K., Yracheta, J., et al. (2020). Rights, interests and expectations: Indigenous perspectives on unrestricted access to genomic data. *Nature Reviews. Genetics, 21*(6), 377–384. https://doi.org/10.1038/s41576-020-0228-x

Israel, T., Farrow, H., Joosten, Y., & Vaughn, Y. (2018) *Community Engagement Studio Toolkit 2.0*. Retrieved from https://victr.vumc.org/wp-content/uploads/2019/07/CESToolkit-2.0.pdf

James, R., Tsosie, R., Sahota, P., Parker, M., Dillard, D., Sylvester, I., et al. (2014). Exploring pathways to trust: A tribal perspective on data sharing. *Genetics in Medicine, 16*(11), 820–826. https://doi.org/10.1038/gim.2014.47

Joosten, Y. A., Israel, T. L., Williams, N. A., Boone, L. R., Schlundt, D. G., Mouton, C. P., et al. (2015). Community engagement studios: A structured approach to obtaining meaningful input from stakeholders to inform research. *Academic Medicine, 90*(12), 1646–1650. https://doi.org/10.1097/acm.0000000000000794

Kennedy, A., Sehgal, A., Szabo, J., McGowan, K., Lindstrom, G., Roach, P., et al. (2022). Indigenous strengths-based approaches to healthcare and health professions education - Recognising the value of elders' teachings. *Health Education Journal, 81*(4), 423–438. https://doi.org/10.1177/00178969221088921

Killough, C. M., Martinez, J., Mata, H., Sedillo, D., Sanjuan, P., Roesch, A., et al. (2024). New horizons in community engagement: Virtual community engagement studios amplifying community voices about health research in New Mexico. *Journal of Clinical and Translational Science, 8*(1), e140. https://doi.org/10.1017/cts.2024.608

Kowalkowski, B., Frieson, L., & Phillips, J. (2022). Community engagement at tribal land-Grant institutions: A tribal approach to reimagining the university-community relationship. *Journal of Community Engagement and Scholarship, 14*(3). https://doi.org/10.54656/jces.v14i3.49

Lafrance, J. (2004). Culturally competent evaluation in Indian country. *New Directions for Evaluation, 2004*, 39–50. https://doi.org/10.1002/ev.114

Lafrance, J., & Nichols, R. (2008). Reframing evaluation: Defining an indigenous evaluation framework. *Canadian Journal of Program Evaluation, 23*, 13–31. https://doi.org/10.3138/cjpe.23.003

Lemke, A. A., Esplin, E. D., Goldenberg, A. J., Gonzaga-Jauregui, C., Hanchard, N. A., Harris-Wai, J., et al. (2022). Addressing underrepresentation in genomics research through community engagement. *American Journal of Human Genetics, 109*(9), 1563–1571. https://doi.org/10.1016/j.ajhg.2022.08.005

Lucero, J. E., Emerson, A. D., Beurle, D., & Roubideaux, Y. (2020). The holding space: A guide for partners in tribal research. *Progress in Community Health Partnerships, 14*(1), 101–107. https://doi.org/10.1353/cpr.2020.0012

Mainous, A. G., 3rd, Kelliher, A., & Warne, D. (2023). Recruiting indigenous patients into clinical trials: A circle of trust. *Annals of Family Medicine, 21*(1), 54–56. https://doi.org/10.1370/afm.2901

Marrero, D. G., Hardwick, E. J., Staten, L. K., Savaiano, D. A., Odell, J. D., Comer, K. F., & Saha, C. (2013). Promotion and tenure for community-engaged research: An examination of promotion and tenure support for community-engaged research at three universities collaborating through a clinical and translational science award. *Clinical and Translational Science, 6*(3), 204–208. https://doi.org/10.1111/cts.12061

Mello, M. M., & Wolf, L. E. (2010). The Havasupai Indian tribe case--lessons for research involving stored biologic samples. *The New England Journal of Medicine, 363*(3), 204–207. https://doi.org/10.1056/NEJMp1005203

Morton, D. J., Proudfit, J., Calac, D., Portillo, M., Lofton-Fitzsimmons, G., Molina, T., et al. (2013). Creating research capacity through a tribally based institutional review board. *American Journal of Public Health, 103*(12), 2160–2164. https://doi.org/10.2105/ajph.2013.301473

Mrklas, K. J., Boyd, J. M., Shergill, S., Merali, S., Khan, M., Nowell, L., et al. (2023). Tools for assessing health research partnership outcomes and impacts: A systematic review. *Health Research Policy and Systems, 21*(1), 3. https://doi.org/10.1186/s12961-022-00937-9

Norström, A. V., Cvitanovic, C., Löf, M. F., West, S., Wyborn, C., Balvanera, P., et al. (2020). Principles for knowledge co-production in sustainability research. *Nature Sustainability, 3*(3), 182–190. https://doi.org/10.1038/s41893-019-0448-2

Pacheco, C. M., Daley, S. M., Brown, T., Filippi, M., Greiner, K. A., & Daley, C. M. (2013). Moving forward: Breaking the cycle of mistrust between American Indians and researchers. *American Journal of Public Health, 103*(12), 2152–2159. https://doi.org/10.2105/ajph.2013.301480

Partners, M. S. I. (2025). *i3 Accelerator*. Retrieved from https://ip.mountsinai.org/i3-accelerator/

Redvers, N., Larson, S., Rajpathy, O., & Olson, D. (2024). American Indian and Alaska native recruitment strategies for health-related randomized controlled trials: A scoping review. *PLoS One, 19*(4), e0302562. https://doi.org/10.1371/journal.pone.0302562

Saunkeah, B., Beans, J. A., Peercy, M. T., Hiratsuka, V. Y., & Spicer, P. (2021). Extending research protections to tribal communities. *The American Journal of Bioethics, 21*(10), 5–12. https://doi.org/10.1080/15265161.2020.1865477

Strickland, C. J. (2006). Challenges in community-based participatory research implementation: Experiences in cancer prevention with Pacific northwest American Indian tribes. *Cancer Control, 13*(3), 230–236. https://doi.org/10.1177/107327480601300312

Thomas, T. W., Hooker, S. A., & Schmittdiel, J. A. (2024). Principles for stakeholder engagement in observational Health Research. *JAMA Health Forum, 5*(3), e240114–e240114. https://doi.org/10.1001/jamahealthforum.2024.0114

Trinidad, S. B., Blacksher, E., Woodbury, R. B., Hopkins, S. E., Burke, W., Woodahl, E. L., et al. (2022). Precision medicine research with American Indian and Alaska native communities: Results of a deliberative engagement with tribal leaders. *Genetics in Medicine, 24*(3), 622–630. https://doi.org/10.1016/j.gim.2021.11.003

Tsosie, R. (2002). Introduction: Symposium on cultural sovereignty. *Arizona State Law Journal, 34*, 1.

Tsosie, R. L., Wu, K., Grant, A. D., Harrington, J., Chase, S. T., Thomas, A., et al. (2024). A growing willow: The six Rs indigenous research framework—Stories of the native American faculty journey in STEM. *Rural Sociology, 89*(S1), 620–637. https://doi.org/10.1111/ruso.12576

Woodbury, R. B., Beans, J. A., Hiratsuka, V. Y., & Burke, W. (2019a). Data Management in Health-Related Research Involving Indigenous Communities in the United States and Canada: A scoping review. *Frontiers in Genetics, 10*, 942. https://doi.org/10.3389/fgene.2019.00942

Woodbury, R. B., Ketchum, S., Hiratsuka, V. Y., & Spicer, P. (2019b). Health-related participatory research in American Indian and Alaska native communities: A scoping review. *International Journal of Environmental Research and Public Health, 16*(16). https://doi.org/10.3390/ijerph16162969

Woodbury, R. B., Beans, J. A., Wark, K. A., Spicer, P., & Hiratsuka, V. Y. (2020). Community perspectives on communicating about precision medicine in an Alaska native tribal health care system. *Frontiers in Communication, 5*. https://doi.org/10.3389/fcomm.2020.00070

Yarborough, M., Edwards, K., Espinoza, P., Geller, G., Sarwal, A., Sharp, R., & Spicer, P. (2013). Relationships hold the key to trustworthy and productive translational science: Recommendations for expanding community engagement in biomedical research. *Clinical and Translational Science, 6*(4), 310–313. https://doi.org/10.1111/cts.12022

The Science of Visibility: Why Native Hawaiian Cancer Data Matters in Research, Public Health, and Genetics

Maile Taualii

Abstract Native Hawaiians experience some of the highest cancer burdens in the United States, yet remain persistently underrepresented in health data, biomedical research, and genetic studies. This systemic invisibility—rooted in historical misclassification, data aggregation, and exclusion—undermines efforts to reduce cancer disparities and advance health equity. This chapter explores how the lack of disaggregated, culturally grounded data for Native Hawaiians impedes public health strategies, precision medicine, and genomic research. We argue that visibility in data is a scientific imperative: inclusion is critical not only to identify disparities but also to inform effective, community-specific interventions. Native Hawaiians offer unique genetic, environmental, and cultural insights that are essential to understanding cancer risk and treatment response. However, scientific progress is hindered without Indigenous representation in cell lines, pharmacogenomics, and genomic databases. Addressing these inequities requires investment in Native Hawaiian-led research, ethical frameworks for data sovereignty, and a robust, culturally competent Indigenous health research workforce. Community-rooted initiatives are models for reclaiming data and driving systemic change. By centering Native Hawaiian knowledge, leadership, and values in research, we can transform cancer care and advance a broader vision of justice, health, and sovereignty for Indigenous communities.

Keywords Native Hawaiian · Cancer · Data · Research · Justice

ʻO ke kahua ma mua, ma hope ke kūkulu. The site first, and then the building.

Wise sayings, or for Native Hawaiians, ʻōlelo noʻeau, are often utilized by Indigenous Peoples to express cultural knowledge and instructions on how to behave and conduct oneself. The ʻōlelo noʻeau above is number 2459 in a treasured book with over 3000 poetical sayings and is often interpreted as "*Learn all you can, then practice*"

M. Taualii (✉)
Center for Integrated Health Care Research, Hawaii Permanente Medical Group, Honolulu, HI, USA
e-mail: Maile.M.Taualii@kp.org

R. C. Haring (ed.), *Indigenous Genetics, Biobanking, Chemistry, and Cancer Research*, Cancer Health Disparities, https://doi.org/10.1007/978-3-032-17296-9_2

(Puku'i, 1983). The beauty of proverbs and poetic sayings is that they allow for interpretation by the user and receiver. I would like to offer a new interpretation; the site or foundation in science is data, and without data, we are unable to describe the challenges, needs, and even successes of our community. This chapter explores the current state of cancer epidemiology among Native Hawaiians and argues there is an urgent need for accurate, disaggregated data that can serve as a cornerstone for equitable health policy and practice.

1 Introduction

Native Hawaiians, the Indigenous people of Hawai'i, face a unique and disproportionate burden of cancer compared with many other racial and ethnic groups in the United States (Haque et al., 2023). While strides have been made in cancer prevention and treatment nationally, Native Hawaiians continue to experience higher incidence and mortality rates for several cancers. A significant factor contributing to these disparities is the persistent invisibility of Native Hawaiians in national health data—a challenge rooted in historical undercounting, misclassification, and aggregation into Asian/Pacific Islanders, despite the 1997 Federal guidelines (Haque et al., 2023). In the age of precision medicine, where treatments are increasingly tailored based on a person's genetic, environmental, and lifestyle profiles, one fact remains painfully true: Native Hawaiians continue to be left out of the data. While this exclusion is most visible in national health statistics and epidemiology, its consequences extend deep into the foundational layers of biomedical research—including basic science, chemistry, and genetics. The lack of robust, disaggregated cancer data for Native Hawaiians undermines not only public health policy but also the advancement of scientific knowledge that could benefit Indigenous communities.

2 Cancer Burden in Native Hawaiian Populations

The limited data available on cancer affecting Native Hawaiians demonstrate that these people experience a disproportionate burden of disease in comparison with many other racial and ethnic groups in the United States. State of Hawai'i data, where only 47% of the Native Hawaiian population resides, highlight numerous cancer disparities among the population (U.S. Census Bureau, 2020; Hawai'i State Department of Health, 2025). Notably, Native Hawaiians suffer from significantly elevated rates of multiple cancers. For example:

- *Liver cancer*: Native Hawaiian men are 2.4 times more likely than non-Hispanic whites to develop liver cancer (Miller et al., 2008)

- *Stomach cancer*: Native Hawaiian men are 2.4 times and Native Hawaiian women are 3.3 times more likely to die of stomach cancer compared to non-Hispanic whites (Miller et al., 2008)
- *Lung cancer*: Although Hawai'i had among the lowest rates of lung cancer in the United States in 2012–2016, lung cancer incidence was highest among Native Hawaiian men and women, and lung cancer mortality was highest in Native Hawaiian women compared to the other population groups in the state (University of Hawai'i Cancer Center, 2016).

These disparities are linked to a range of social determinants, including poverty, lower access to preventive screenings, environmental exposures, and systemic racism in healthcare delivery. Native Hawaiians often present with more aggressive disease at younger ages and have lower survival rates than their white and Asian counterparts. For example, Native Hawaiians had the highest mortality rate (404.8) for all types of cancer, as compared to whites (136.5) in Hawai'i 2013–2015 (Hawai'i State Department of Health, 2025). Nationally, Native Hawaiian and Pacific Islanders had the highest cancer death rates among 20–49-year-olds (43.7/100,000) compared to all races (Haque et al., 2023).

3 Challenges in Data Collection and Representation

Data challenges are central to the persistence of these disparities. Key problems include:

- *Racial misclassification*: Studies have shown that Native Hawaiians are frequently misclassified as "Other" or as part of the "Asian and Pacific Islander (API)" umbrella in medical records and national datasets. Misclassification rates in cancer registries may be as high as 10–20% (Arias et al., 2016).
- *Data aggregation*: Grouping Native Hawaiians with other Pacific Islanders, such as Samoans or Tongans, obscures important intragroup differences. For instance, while both groups may experience health disparities, the epidemiological profiles, genetic factors, and cultural contexts differ significantly, warranting separate analysis.
- *Sample size issues*: National surveys such as the Behavioral Risk Factor Surveillance System (BRFSS) and National Health Interview Survey (NHIS) often yield insufficient Native Hawaiian samples for statistically valid subgroup analyses.

The statement "If you're not counted, you don't count. And if you don't count, you don't get the resources" highlights the crucial link between being included in national health reporting and receiving essential resources. It emphasizes that without being part of the counted population, individuals and communities may not receive the support they need, whether it is access to programs, funding, or services. This invisibility in data perpetuates a cycle of neglect in funding, research priorities, and policy development. Without accurate epidemiological profiles, public health interventions may be inappropriately designed, leading to limited effectiveness.

4 Why Data Representation in Basic Science Matters

Basic science—the foundational study of cells, molecules, and biochemical processes—drives innovation in cancer detection and treatment. However, most of this work relies on data collected from majority populations (National Academies of Sciences, Engineering, and Medicine, 2022).

Cell lines and tissue repositories: In cancer biology, human-derived cell lines are critical for understanding tumor behavior and testing drugs. Yet, there is a stark underrepresentation of Native Hawaiian-derived biological samples in national repositories such as the Cancer Genome Atlas (National Cancer Institutes, 2025). Without Native Hawaiian inclusion or any unique community being represented, there is a risk of missing:

- Unique genetic mutations that may influence cancer development or drug resistance.
- Environmental exposures that interact with cellular pathways in ways specific to Native Hawaiian communities.
- Tumor microenvironment features potentially shaped by ancestry and diet.

This absence leads to a cascade of missed opportunities in translational science, making it harder to identify risk markers or effective treatments specific to Native Hawaiians.

At the chemical level, cancer is a disease of disrupted signaling—proteins misfold, enzymes malfunction, and DNA repair mechanisms fail. Precision oncology often relies on the identification of specific biomolecular targets, such as overexpressed receptors or mutated enzymes.

Pharmacogenomics and drug metabolism: Genetic ancestry influences how the body metabolizes drugs. Native Hawaiians, who often have mixed Polynesian and Asian ancestry, may carry unique allelic variants affecting:

- Cytochrome P450 enzymes, key players in metabolizing chemotherapy agents.
- Transporter proteins, which affect drug absorption and toxicity.
- DNA repair genes, influencing how effectively a tumor responds to radiation or alkylating agents.

A lack of Native Hawaiian representation in pharmacogenomic databases leads to assumptions that therapies effective in other populations will work similarly—an assumption that can increase adverse reactions or therapeutic failure.

5 Genetics, Ancestry, and Cancer Risk

Genetic predisposition is a growing area of cancer research. Hereditary cancer syndromes such as BRCA1/2 (linked to breast and ovarian cancer) are well-documented in European populations, but few studies have mapped these or other high-risk genes among Native Hawaiians.

Underrepresentation in genomic studies: Large-scale genome-wide association studies (GWAS) have disproportionately focused on individuals of European descent. According to a 2019 review in *Cell*, over 78% of participants in GWAS studies are of European ancestry (Peterson et al., 2019).

This means:

- Gene–environment interactions specific to Pacific populations remain unexplored.
- Variants of unknown significance (VUS) in Native Hawaiian genomes may go unclassified, delaying clinical action.
- The development of polygenic risk scores (PRS) that guide screening and prevention are less accurate or applicable for Native Hawaiians.

Mitochondrial and epigenetic markers: Emerging research into mitochondrial DNA and epigenetic modifications shows that population-specific factors (such as diet, stress, and cultural trauma) can affect cancer risk across generations. Without dedicated Native Hawaiian cohorts, these studies either ignore Indigenous biology or apply potentially misleading conclusions.

5.1 Case Example: Breast Cancer in Native Hawaiian Women

Native Hawaiians had the lowest percentage of breast cancer diagnosed with localized stage (61.9%) and highest percentage diagnosed at the advanced stage (35.2%) (Loo et al., 2019). These trends in the distribution of stage of diagnosis across the major racial and/or ethnic groups have persisted for more than 15 years. This discrepancy is often attributed to late-stage diagnosis, but deeper questions remain:

- Are tumors biologically different in Native Hawaiian women?
- Could unique mutations or receptor expressions affect how the disease progresses or responds to therapy?
- Are screening guidelines, based on studies of white women, insufficiently sensitive for Native Hawaiians?

Without access to molecular-level data (e.g., tumor subtypes, gene mutations), these questions remain unanswered. Investing in community-driven genomic research could illuminate these blind spots.

6 Weighing the Benefits and Risks of Research

What is unique to Native Hawaiians and all Indigenous Peoples is that there are collective risks and harms to participating in research. Recent and historical abuses of Indigenous Peoples have made participation in research a potential risky endeavor. While the majority of population research participants may weigh the risks to their individual person, Indigenous Peoples also face collective harm that could put their legal rights at risk (Garrison et al., 2019).

In addition to mistrust stemming from historical and recent unethical research practices and exploitation, many research protocols lack culturally grounded consent processes that honor community values. Some research protocols, including very large national efforts, lacked community consenting, circumnavigating members of the Native Hawaiian community, who walk in both the research world and cultural spaces. The edge walkers are both Native Hawaiian scientists and cultural practitioners who can help to bring Native Hawaiian leaders to the table to consider the risks and benefits of participating in research. Informed consent depends on all aspects of the research processes to be considered, including risks to legal, traditional, and customary practices.

Native Hawaiian-led organizations have developed ethical frameworks that prioritize data sovereignty—thereby ensuring that community's control how their biological and genetic information is used (Halmai et al., 2025). These include Community Review Boards for research proposals, benefit-sharing models that guarantee findings are translated into local health improvements, and the integration of cultural protocols in the handling of biological specimens.

7 Community-Based Data Sovereignty and Leadership

Efforts led by Native Hawaiian organizations and scholars are making strides in reclaiming and reshaping the narrative around health data. Key initiatives include:

- *'Imi Hale—Native Hawaiian Cancer Network*: A community-based participatory research (CBPR) model that emphasizes Indigenous values in cancer education, prevention, and data collection. This group has trained over 100 Native Hawaiian researchers and conducted culturally adapted interventions (Santos et al., 2001).
- *Papa Ola Lōkahi*: Advocates for Native Hawaiian health by coordinating research, data systems, and policy across communities and healthcare providers. Their work supports the development of Native Hawaiian Health Indicators—a vital tool for local accountability.

These models exemplify how data sovereignty—the right of Indigenous Peoples to govern the collection, ownership, and application of their own data—can be a powerful force for change.

8 Building a Native Hawaiian Research Workforce: Beyond Discovery to Justice

The absence of Native Hawaiian participants in basic cancer science is not just an issue of fairness, it is a scientific failure. Precision medicine, drug discovery, and genomics are all advanced by diverse, inclusive datasets. Native Hawaiians offer genetic diversity that can reveal novel mechanisms of disease, a unique history that can inform environmental carcinogenesis, and cultural practices that can shape epigenetic expression, yielding insights into how social context affects biology. Without these voices and bodies in the laboratory, cancer research will remain incomplete—and cancer disparities will persist.

Representation and inclusion go well beyond research participants and discovery. Native Hawaiians remain underrepresented in biomedical research and among the professionals conducting it. Cultivating a health research workforce drawn from the Native Hawaiian community is vital for culturally grounded, community-engaged, and equity-focused research. A critical step toward health equity is developing a robust Native Hawaiian health research workforce that can lead, conduct, and disseminate research with cultural integrity and community accountability.

The marginalization of Native Hawaiians in health and science cannot be separated from the broader history of colonization, land dispossession, and systemic erasure. Research historically conducted *on* Native communities rather than *with* them has contributed to mistrust and low participation in clinical studies (Gray et al., 2013). Additionally, Western biomedical models often fail to account for Indigenous worldviews, such as the holistic Native Hawaiian concept of health (*ola*) that includes physical, emotional, spiritual, and environmental well-being. This disconnect reduces participation in research studies and undermines the effectiveness of interventions developed without genuine community input.

Native Hawaiians are underrepresented in health professions and research careers, accounting for only about 0.4% of US physicians and even fewer NIH-funded researchers (AAMC, 2019; National Institutes of Health, 2025). Without Native Hawaiian researchers at the table, data gaps persist, culturally relevant questions go unasked, and health inequities remain poorly addressed.

Researchers who share cultural heritage with participants are more likely to approach communities with cultural humility, fluency in local values (e.g., *kuleana*, *pono*), and deeper empathy. Native Hawaiian researchers bring ʻike (knowledge), language, and cultural fluency essential for building trust and engaging communities. Trust is foundational for research participation, particularly in communities with a history of colonization and scientific exploitation (Taualii et al., 2014). Researchers from Native Hawaiian communities are more likely to pursue questions relevant to their people, including the role of ʻāina (land), moʻomeheu (culture), and pilina (relationships) in health and healing. These questions might otherwise be overlooked by non-Native researchers. Community-rooted researchers are more attuned to ethical nuances and culturally safe methods, enhancing the accuracy, relevance, and acceptability of research (Look et al., 2023). Initiatives like *ʻImi*

Hale—Native Hawaiian Cancer Network have shown the success of culturally grounded, community-driven research models in improving participation and outcomes (Santos et al., 2001). Culturally competent researchers play a crucial role in disaggregating data and advocating for more accurate and meaningful reporting (Brach & Fraser, 2000). Training Native Hawaiians in health research contributes to long-term community resilience, supports educational and economic opportunity, and cultivates future leaders committed to *lāhui* (nationhood and collective well-being). Investing in Native Hawaiian researchers fosters leadership in health sciences and contributes to broader self-determination in health policy and practice. It also serves as a form of social justice and reparation.

9 Future Directions and Policy Recommendations

Listing all the barriers at the root of cancer disparities facing Native Hawaiians can leave one feeling overwhelmed and paralyzed into not knowing where to start. Our community faces extreme challenges, but the flip side of that is that there are a multitude of opportunities to make improvements. This chapter focuses on the challenges with visibility, representation in research studies, warranted distrust of the research process, and a lack of representation in all aspects of the research process. Invisibility in data is a scientific problem—and visibility is a scientific imperative. As we enter the next era of personalized medicine, ensuring that Native Hawaiians are seen, included, engaged, and in control of each step is not optional, it is essential for science, for equity, and for life.

To address the cancer disparities facing Native Hawaiians, the following policy actions are recommended:

1. Fund Indigenous-led genomic and molecular studies, especially in Native Hawaiian and closely related Pacific Islander communities.
2. Create representative cell lines, tissue banks, and biorepositories with appropriate ethical safeguards.
3. Mandate the inclusion and representation of Native Hawaiians in clinical trials and databases.
4. Invest in training Native Hawaiian scientists who can lead this research from within the community.

10 Conclusion

The disproportionate burden of cancer among Native Hawaiians is a symptom of a deeper systemic issue: the ongoing erasure of Indigenous People from the data that drives healthcare decisions. Data visibility is foundational to health equity. It is only through accurate, disaggregated, and community-centered data that the true scope of cancer disparities can be seen—and meaningfully addressed. The fight against cancer in Native Hawaiian communities cannot be won without first recognizing the systemic gaps in data that hinder progress. Visibility in health statistics is not just a technical issue, it is a matter of justice.

Addressing these disparities requires a commitment to collecting disaggregated, accurate, and culturally respectful data; support for Native Hawaiian leadership in research; and development of policies that reflect the lived realities of Indigenous communities. Developing a Native Hawaiian health research workforce is not merely a strategy, it is a necessity for addressing persistent health disparities. By investing in the education, training, and leadership of Native Hawaiians in research, we will build capacity to produce knowledge that is relevant, respectful, and responsive. Such efforts can bridge the long-standing divide between research institutions and Native communities, ultimately advancing health equity and restoring self-determination in health.

Native Hawaiian communities have long understood the power of knowledge rooted in relationships, land, and collective well-being. By centering Indigenous voices in data collection and interpretation, we can not only improve cancer outcomes but also advance a broader vision of justice, health, and sovereignty for all Native Hawaiian people.

As we look to the future, a focus on Indigenous data sovereignty, investment in community-led research, and accountability in public health systems will be critical to achieving health equity and improving cancer outcomes for Native Hawaiians.

Acknowledgments I would like to express my deepest gratitude to the mentors who have guided and supported me throughout this work. Your wisdom, encouragement, and unwavering commitment to Indigenous health equity have profoundly shaped my thinking and strengthened my resolve. You have not only shared your knowledge but also modeled how to lead with integrity, cultural grounding, and a deep sense of kuleana. I am especially thankful for the time you have taken to guide me, challenge my assumptions, and help me navigate both academic and community spaces with care. Mahalo nui for believing in me and for walking alongside me in this journey.

Kuni ʻōlino ke kukui
Ke Mele o nā mamo
Hoʻo Noa iā Kanaloa
Hoʻoulu hua nā Pua i ka lani
E ulana ka naʻauao me he Lei momi la
ʻIke ʻia ke Ala o ka liko
Wili ʻia ka Lei me na lima akahai
Pūliki ka pō, mālamalama nā hōkū
Māhuahua ka maile, paʻa ka maile, oʻo ka Maile

References

AAMC. (2019). *Diversity in medicine: Facts and figures*. https://www.aamc.org/data-reports/workforce/report/diversity-medicine-facts-and-figures-2019

Arias, E., Heron, M., & Hakes, J. (2016). The validity of race and Hispanic-origin reporting on death certificates in the United States: An update. National Center for Health Statistics. *Vital Health Stat, 2*(172), 1–21.

Brach, C., & Fraser, I. (2000). Can cultural competency reduce racial and ethnic health disparities? A review and conceptual model. *Medical Care Research and Review, 57*(Suppl 1), 181–217.

Garrison, N. A., Hudson, M., Ballantyne, L. L., Garba, I., Martinez, A., Taualii, M., Arbour, L., Caron, N. R., & Rainie, S. C. (2019). Genomic research through an indigenous lens: Understanding the expectations. *Annual Review of Genomics and Human Genetics, 20*, 495–517.

Gray, M., Coates, J., Yellow Bird, M., & Hetherington, T. (Eds.). (2013). *Decolonizing social work* (1st ed.). Routledge. Chapter 22. Matsuoka, J. K., Morelli P. T., McCubbin, H. Indigenizing Research for Culturally Relevant Social Work Practice.

Halmai, N. B., Taitingfong, R., Jennings, L. L., Yracheta, J., Garba, I., Lund, J. R., Curley, C. A., Claw, K. G., Taualii, M., Garrison, N. A., & Carroll, S. R. (2025). Indigenous data sovereignty in genomics and human genetics: Genomic equity and justice for indigenous peoples. *Annual Review of Genomics and Human Genetics, 18*. https://doi.org/10.1146/annurev-genom-022024-125543

Haque, A. T., Berrington de González, A., Chen, Y., Haozous, E. A., Inoue-Choi, M., Lawrence, W. R., McGee-Avila, J. K., Nápoles, A. M., Pérez-Stable, E. J., Taparra, K., & Vo, J. B. (2023). Cancer mortality rates by racial and ethnic groups in the United States, 2018–2020. *JNCI: Journal of the National Cancer Institute, 115*(7), 822–830.

Hawaii State Department of Health. (2025). *Hawai'i Health Data warehouse database search results* ["Native Hawaiian" on July 20, 2025] Honolulu, Hawaii. Available from https://hhdw.org/

Loo, L. W. M., Williams, M., & Hernandez, B. Y. (2019). The high and heterogeneous burden of breast cancer in Hawaii: A unique multiethnic U.S. population. *Cancer Epidemiology, 58*, 71–76.

Look, M. A., Maskarinec, G. G., de Silva, M., Werner, K., Mabellos, T., Palakiko, D. M., Haumea, S. L., Gonsalves, J., Seabury, A. A., Vegas, J. K., Solatorio, C., & Kaholokula, J. K. (2023). Developing culturally-responsive health promotion: Insights from cultural experts. *Health Promotion International, 38*(2), daad022.

Miller, B. A., Chu, K. C., Hankey, B. F., & Ries, L. A. G. (2008). Cancer incidence and mortality patterns among specific Asian and Pacific islander populations in the U.S. *Cancer Causes Control, 19*(3), 227–256.

National Academies of Sciences, Engineering, and Medicine. (2022). Policy and global affairs; committee on women in science, engineering, and medicine; committee on improving the representation of women and underrepresented minorities in clinical trials and research. In K. Bibbins-Domingo & A. Helman (Eds.), *Improving representation in clinical trials and research: Building research equity for women and underrepresented groups* (Vol. 2). National Academies Press (US). Why Diverse Representation in Clinical Research Matters and the Current State of Representation within the Clinical Research Ecosystem.

National Cancer Institute. (2025). *Genomic data commons, data portal. Database search results* [race cohort "native Hawaiian"]. Accessed 20 July 2025. National Institutes of Health.

National Institutes of Health (2025). *NIH RePORTER database search results* [on "Native Hawaiian" on April 10, 2025]. National Institutes of Health. Available from: https://reporter.nih.gov

Peterson, R. E., et al. (2019). Genome-wide association studies in ancestrally diverse populations: Opportunities, methods, pitfalls, and recommendations. *Cell, 179*(3), 589–603. https://doi.org/10.1016/j.cell.2019.08.051

Puku'i, M. K. (1983). *Ōlelo No'eau: Hawaiian proverbs and poetical sayings*. Bishop Museum Press.

Santos, L., Mokuau, N., Abrigo, L., Braun, K. L., Tsark, J. U., Mackura, G., Kuhaulua, R., & Chong, C. D. (2001). Imi Hale: Establishing an inheritance for native Hawaiians on cancer awareness, research and training. *Pacific Health Dialog, 8*(2), 436–445.

Taualii, M., Davis, E. L., Braun, K. L., Tsark, J. U., Brown, N., Hudson, M., & Burke, W. (2014). Native Hawaiian views on biobanking. *Journal of Cancer Education, 29*(3), 570–576. Erratum in: J Cancer Educ. 2020 Feb;35(1):210.

U.S. Census Bureau. (2020). *Race and ethnicity*. https://data.census.gov/table/DECENNIALDHC2020.P8?g=010XX00US. Accessed 15 Apr 2025.

University of Hawai'i Cancer Center. (2016). *Hawai'i Cancer at a Glance 2012–2016*. Accessed 20 July 2025. https://www.uhcancercenter.org/pdf/htr/Hawaii%20Cancer%20at%20a%20Glance%202012_2016.pdf

The Microbiome, Cancer, and Health Disparities: Implications for Native American Communities in the Southwest

Krystal Charley, Nicole Jimenez, Paweł Łaniewski, Melissa Herbst-Kralovetz, Emily Cope, Fernando Monroy, Jani Ingram, and Naomi Lee

Keywords Two-eyed seeing · HPV · *H. pylori* · Immunotherapies · Partnership for Native American Cancer Prevention (NACP)

1 Introduction: An Indigenous Perspective on the Microbiome

The human microbiome consists of a diverse array of bacteria, viruses, fungi, protozoa, and archaea found throughout the body. Most of these microbes are harmless and contribute to essential bodily processes, helping to maintain homeostasis by supporting biological functions and preventing the overgrowth of harmful microbes (Lloyd-Price et al., 2016). The composition of the microbiome can be influenced by

K. Charley · J. Ingram · N. Lee (✉)
Department of Chemistry and Biochemistry, Partnership for Native American Cancer Prevention, Northern Arizona University, Flagstaff, AZ, USA
e-mail: Krystal.Charley@nau.edu; Jani.ingram@nau.edu; naomi.lee@nau.edu

N. Jimenez
Department of Obstetrics and Gynecology, Partnership for Native American Cancer Prevention, University of Arizona College of Medicine–Phoenix, Phoenix, AZ, USA
e-mail: nicolejimenez@arizona.edu

P. Łaniewski
Department of Basic Medical Sciences, Partnership for Native American Cancer Prevention, University of Arizona College of Medicine–Phoenix, Phoenix, AZ, USA
e-mail: laniewski@arizona.edu

M. Herbst-Kralovetz
Department of Basic Medical Sciences, Department of Obstetrics and Gynecology, Partnership for Native American Cancer Prevention, University of Arizona College of Medicine–Phoenix, Phoenix, AZ, USA
e-mail: mherbst1@arizona.edu

R. C. Haring (ed.), *Indigenous Genetics, Biobanking, Chemistry, and Cancer Research*, Cancer Health Disparities, https://doi.org/10.1007/978-3-032-17296-9_3

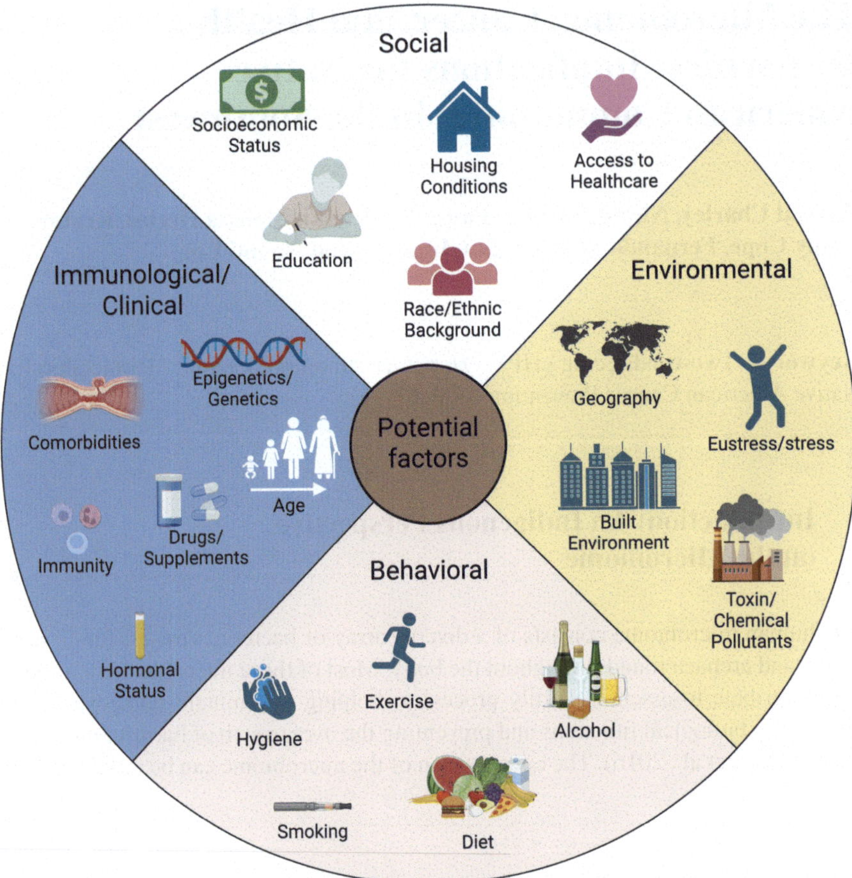

Fig. 1 Factors that can impact the microbiome and the host that increase the risk of cancer. The microbiome is influenced by a variety of factors, regardless of the type of cancer. These factors can be categorized as follows: (1) Social factors (e.g., access to healthcare can be challenging for some Indigenous communities). (2) Environmental factors (e.g., responses to eustress or stress can impact health). (3) Immunological and clinical factors (e.g., effective or ineffective immune response to pathogens and tumors). (4) Behavioral factors (e.g., diet and exercise can have a significant impact on health). Many of these factors can either positively or negatively impact well-being and the microbiome. (The figure was created using Biorender and is adapted from Morales et al. (2022))

E. Cope
Department of Biological Sciences, Pathogen and Microbiome Institute, Partnership for Native American Cancer Prevention, Northern Arizona University, Flagstaff, AZ, USA
e-mail: Emily.cope@nau.edu

F. Monroy
Department of Biological Sciences, Partnership for Native American Cancer Prevention, Northern Arizona University, Flagstaff, AZ, USA
e-mail: fernanado.monroy@nau.edu

factors such as lifestyle, diet, environment, and overall health (Fig. 1). Many tribes such as the Navajo (Diné) embrace a similar core cultural concept known as "Walk in beauty" and living "Hozho," which emphasizes the importance of balance and harmony within oneself, with others and the surroundings (Kahn-John Diné & Koithan, 2015). Another example of this concept is also reflected in the Hopi beliefs where the way of life revolves around harmony with Nature and all in the universe is sacred and interconnected. Within each person, this balance includes both good and bad cells, as well as beneficial and harmful microbes that coexist in the body.

Box 1 Use of Terms

Please note the distinctions between terms used to describe our population of study. Native American is a broader description of both urban and reservation-based American Indians. American Indian and Alaska Natives (AI/ANs), a political term that recognizes First Americans, is the description that is used by federal agencies, including research and census entities. The Tribes/Tribal designation is reserved for federally recognized sovereign nations, and urban organizations do not use it. Indian Country is the collective of Native communities in the United States. Depending on the context, these terms are used as appropriate within the chapter.

Disruption of the body's "balance and harmony," particularly concerning the microbiome, can increase the risk of cancer. Studies show that an imbalanced microbiome can lead to various health issues that heighten cancer risk (Lim, 2025). For instance, since Native American populations began assimilating into White societal ways, their diets have changed significantly. There is now a higher consumption of processed foods high in fat, along with more sedentary lifestyles, which have negatively impacted the gut microbiome. These changes have been linked to increased rates of obesity, health problems, and cancers among Native Americans, likely due to this microbiome imbalance (Story et al., 1999). Certain gut microbes, such as *Helicobacter pylori*, *Bacteroides fragilis*, *Fusobacterium nucleatum*, *Faecalibacterium praunsnitzii*, and *Akkermansia muciniphila*, have been associated with a higher cancer risk. This is mainly due to the toxins produced by these microbes that promote DNA damage and inflammation (Lim, 2025). Conversely, a reduction in beneficial microbes, such as those that produce tumor-suppressing metabolites from dietary fiber, has been shown to elevate cancer risk (Singh et al., 2023). Given that these imbalances are linked to cancers, the microbiome is a critical factor in cancer prevention and treatment. Restoring balance in the body can involve various strategies, including ceremonial practices and Western medicines, as well as preventive approaches that rely on community health advocacy. Many tribes utilize both cultural ceremonies and Western medicines to treat illnesses, including cancers. In the following sections, we will discuss ideas and ongoing projects that emphasize the microbiome and its connection to health, prevention, and treatment strategies, while incorporating Indigenous perspectives.

2 Introduction to Cancer Health Disparities in Native American Communities

Cancer impacts all racial and ethnic groups. However, the impact varies by cancer type, region, gender, and mortality rate within the United States (U.S.) (Burhansstipanov et al., 2022). From 2015 to 2019, American Indian and Alaska Natives (AI/AN) had an 18% higher mortality rate compared to non-Hispanic Whites (NHW) (CDC, 2023a). Despite the variations of cancer types, the microbiome is believed to play a significant role in cancer progression (Laniewski et al., 2020b; Lythgoe et al., 2022; Sepich-Poore et al., 2021). Risk of cancer and the microbiome are both influenced by behavioral, environmental, social, clinical, and immunological factors that impact cancer screenings, detection, and treatment (Fig. 1) (Morales et al., 2022). In addition to the known factors, AI/AN communities experience unique factors that increase cancer and other health disparities; these include the rooted distrust with researchers, healthcare providers, and the federal government (Bordeaux et al., 2021).

When conducting research in AI/AN communities, it is important to note that additional reviews and approvals, e.g., universities and tribal IRBs, are often required, varying from tribe to tribe. Many tribes have established their own Institutional Review Boards (IRBs), which must be considered alongside university IRB approvals (Morton et al., 2013). Tribal IRBs typically include members of the tribal council, providing valuable perspective and input from tribal leaders. Additionally, communities may require approval from the IRB associated with the regional or national Indian Health Services (IHS). These IHS IRBs may oversee multiple tribes, such as those in the Southwestern region. Navigating the IRB processes can be complex for researchers who may not fully understand the sovereignty and historical traumas that AI/AN communities have experienced.

The partnership for Native American Cancer Prevention (NACP), through a collaboration between the University of Arizona Cancer Center (UACC) and Northern Arizona University (NAU), is dedicated to addressing cancer disparities and supporting researchers working with AI/AN communities across the southwest U.S. NACP is currently a 22-year collaboration between the two universities that has been recently renewed for continued growth with Native American communities. Over the years, NACP has made significant strides in addressing the factors that contribute to cancer inequities among AI/AN populations through its work with sovereign tribal nations in Arizona and beyond. Additionally, NACP has positively impacted the career pathways of AI/AN individuals interested in cancer health and research by training early- and mid-stage Native investigators who are becoming leaders in this field. Moreover, NACP has driven institutional change at both NAU and UACC by increasing cancer research capacity at NAU and promoting health disparity-focused research at UACC. The partnership has also strengthened both institutions' commitments to serving AI/AN students and communities. NACP has built a strong foundation of relationships with tribal communities, governments, and other partners based on trust and respect, resulting in an accelerated positive impact from its initiatives.

Over the years, the NACP has supported research projects focused on various types of cancer, including stomach/gastric cancer, breast cancer, liver cancer, colorectal cancer, prostate cancer, and cervical cancer. Among AI/AN women in Arizona, breast cancer is the most frequently diagnosed type of cancer and is responsible for the highest number of cancer-related deaths compared to other types. Additionally, a comparison between AI/AN in Arizona and NHW reveals that AI/AN experience disproportionately higher rates of prostate, kidney, gastric, ovarian, endometrial, and cervical cancers (Gachupin et al., 2021). Recently, NACP introduced an intellectual and operational framework designed to systematically incorporate Indigenous perspectives as a core reference in its work. Specifically, NACP embraces the "two-eyed seeing" paradigm (Fig. 2) (Martin, 2012) that seeks to "*see from one eye with the strengths of Indigenous knowledges and ways of knowing, and from the other eye with the strengths of Western knowledges and ways of knowing, and to use both of these eyes together for the benefit of all.*" This guiding principle provides NACP with an overarching framework that we apply consistently throughout the entire partnership, with the support of our AI/AN community partners.

The chapter starts by outlining various therapeutic approaches to address the immune system and microbiome. The application of the approaches may guide healthcare professionals in addressing cancer that work in AI/AN communities. In addition, we will highlight two NACP projects that utilize the "two-eyed seeing" paradigm to implement cultural concepts for methodologies, cultivate trust between collaborators, gain Indigenous perspectives on research findings, and address specific challenges, such as distrust in scientific research among participating

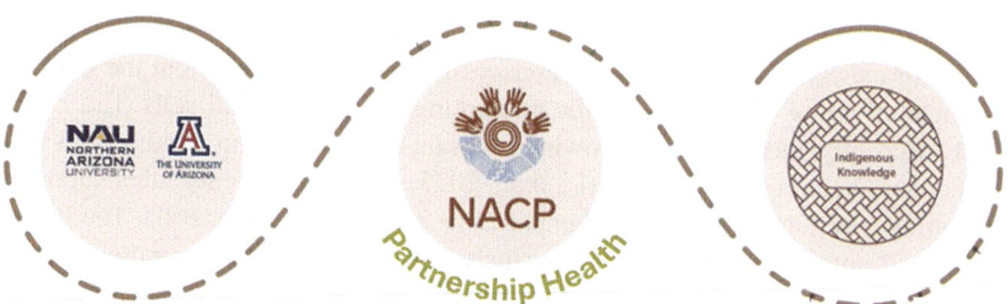

Fig. 2 NACP embraces the "two-eyed seeing" paradigm. In the research projects, the concept of two-eyed seeing is applied through the engagement, input, and perspectives of AI/AN communities. This approach combines traditional knowledge with Western scientific methods, such as bench science, to address questions related to cancer biomedicine. The integration of these methods aims to address health disparities within Indigenous populations

communities and obstacles researchers encounter with university and tribal IRB processes. One of the projects focuses on the role of *Helicobacter pylori* (*H. pylori*) and the gut microbiome as a risk factor for gastric cancer among the Navajo people. The second project investigates the relationship between human papillomavirus (HPV), the vaginal microbiome, and cervical cancer among AI/AN women in Arizona. Both projects also examine significant factors associated with the microbiome (Fig. 1) (Kandalai et al., 2023). Globally, studies have been conducted on Indigenous communities; however, the heterogeneity of these groups necessitates more focused evaluations to address the specific cancer needs of AI/AN populations in the U.S. (Sankaranarayanan et al., 2015; Warbrick et al., 2023). Therefore, the book chapter aims to provide an overview of stomach cancer caused by *H. pylori* and the gastric microbiome, as well as cervical cancer linked to HPV and the vaginal microbiome. The discussions will focus on various AI/AN populations located in the southwestern U.S.

3 Balance: Therapeutic Approaches with the Immune System and Microbiome

AI/AN populations are more likely to receive cancer diagnoses at later stages and more advanced levels of the disease (Holt et al., 2023). Therefore, it is important to investigate effective prevention and treatment strategies for cancer within AI/AN and other underrepresented communities. Furthermore, many underrepresented groups, including AI/ANs and Hispanics, often lack sufficient information about available preventive healthcare and treatment options (Guadagnolo et al., 2017). As a result, it is essential to examine these disparities in AI/AN communities to improve research and healthcare while respecting their cultural and traditional beliefs and practices. Such studies require collaboration and support, particularly from AI/AN perspectives and AI/AN-led research. Programs such as NACP (Fig. 2) can help increase the participation of AI/AN individuals and support underrepresented students and investigators in the cancer biomedical field.

Chemotherapy and radiation therapy have traditionally been the standard treatments for cancer. Both methods are nonspecific and work throughout the body to eliminate dividing cancer cells while attempting to spare normal cells (Liu et al., 2021). Recently, there has been growing focus on developing immunotherapies that target tumors and related diseases (Li et al., 2023). These treatments either suppress the immune system or activate and enhance its response to tumor cells. The tumor microenvironment surrounding a tumor includes various responding immune cells, which can become dysregulated due to signals emitted by tumor cells. This dysregulation allows tumors to evade immune surveillance and suppress the immune system (Vinay et al., 2015). However, immunotherapies have the potential to reshape the tumor microenvironment, helping restore the immune system's ability to eliminate tumors effectively (Lv et al., 2022).

3.1 Immunotherapies

Immune checkpoint therapy is a form of immunotherapy that targets checkpoint molecules, which are often upregulated by tumor cells. Immune checkpoint inhibitors (ICIs) such as CTLA-4 and PD-1 inhibitors have been used to treat various cancers (Rotte, 2019). These checkpoint molecules are expressed by immune cells and play a crucial role in regulating immune tolerance and responses at different stages (He & Xu, 2020). ICIs are promising treatments that enhance the patient's immune system ability to eliminate tumor cells. While treatment with single ICIs has shown improvement in immune response, combination therapy may be recommended when monotherapy is ineffective, especially in the case of aggressive cancers. Using more than one ICI in combination can potentially lead to better antitumor responses than single-agent therapy (Hellmann et al., 2017). However, ICIs can significantly alter immune responses, leading to increased side effects that can present additional challenges. Moreover, some cancer patients do not respond to either single or combination therapy with ICIs. The reasons for this lack of response are complex, as the effectiveness of the immune response depends on both the characteristics of the tumor and the patient's immune system. For instance, some tumors have a higher mutational burden, which complicates treatment due to the presence of multiple antigens or markers. Conversely, patients may initially respond to treatment but later develop resistance to single or combination immunotherapy (Pandey & Ernstoff, 2019). Additionally, studies have reported cases of immune-related adverse events (irAEs), which are side effects associated with the use of ICIs, particularly in combination therapies. These events can lead to dysfunction, toxicity, and the development of autoimmune conditions at any stage of treatment (Yin et al., 2023). Given these complexities, it is crucial to understand the risks associated with anticancer treatments such as ICIs, especially in underrepresented and understudied populations, such as AI/AN and non-White Hispanics, where the use and effectiveness of cancer immunotherapies may be limited.

Adoptive cellular therapy is another form of immunotherapy worth considering. This approach uses the patient's own immune cells to target cancer and other diseases. The process involves collecting immune cells directly from the patient, which can then be genetically modified, expanded, and reintroduced into the patient's body to help control infections or tumors (Du et al., 2023). It is important to note that adoptive cell therapy requires a functional immune response, so patients with immunosuppression may not benefit from it. While there are potential challenges such as toxicity and off-target effects, adoptive cell therapy is generally considered less toxic than some other forms of immunotherapy and can promote a more targeted immune response (June, 2007). A well-known example of approved adoptive cellular therapies is chimeric antigen receptor (CAR) T cell therapy. In this method, T cells are acquired from the patient and genetically engineered to recognize specific antigens associated with the target cancer or pathogen. Although CAR T cell therapy is relatively new and primarily used to treat blood cancers, research is ongoing for its application in solid tumors (Feng et al., 2022; Yu et al., 2023). Because this therapy utilizes the patient's own cells, AI/AN and other underrepresented groups may be more inclined to accept it, as it is generally nontoxic and, depending on the specific tribe, may not be perceived as foreign. Nonetheless, ongoing improvements in adoptive cell therapy aim to enhance its effectiveness. Including AI/AN populations in clinical trials and studies for adoptive cellular therapies is essential for advancing its efficacy and relevance (Emole et al., 2022).

3.2 *Vaccines*

Research on vaccines targeting oncogenic pathogens and tumor cells is an important area in the fight against cancer (Lin et al., 2022). These vaccines are designed using antigen derived from either the pathogen or tumor cells to stimulate an immune response. The memory immune cells produced after vaccination protects patients from subsequent infections or tumor cells (Lin et al., 2022). Anticancer vaccines show great promise in preventing cancer development and progression; however, neoantigens, which are new antigens arising from a high tumor mutational burden, can pose challenges (Xie et al., 2023). Additionally, cancer-causing pathogens, such as certain viruses, can have multiple strains that present differential antigens and exhibit varying effects on the host. Therefore, it is essential to design vaccines that incorporate multiple and diverse antigens to ensure broad coverage. This approach is especially important for preventing infections linked to oncogenic pathogens, such as HPV, particularly in underrepresented communities where oncogenic HPV types are prevalent. Additionally, the prevalence of different oncogenic HPV types varies across geographical regions and populations, highlighting another critical gap that needs further investigation. Recent efforts to include AI/AN in clinical trials and studies demonstrate progress in addressing health and educational disparities related to infectious diseases and cancer. It is essential to continue prioritizing the inclusion of AI/AN individuals in vaccine trials and to promote education about anticancer vaccines (Bordeaux et al., 2021).

3.3 *Microbiome*

The human microbiome consists of commensal microorganisms that play a crucial role in the development and functioning of the immune system. The microbiome is incredibly diverse and forms a complex system characterized by various symbiotic relationships between the microbiota and host cells, including immune cells. The microbiota helps protect and stabilize the human body, contributing to maintenance of homeostasis (Li et al., 2024). The establishment of the microbiome begins early, during and after childbirth, primarily influenced by the maternal microbiome and the surrounding environment (Amir et al., 2020; Huang et al., 2014; Zheng et al., 2020). Specifically, the newborn acquires its microbiota from the mother, and this process initiates the education of the newborn's own microbiome and immune system immediately after birth. Initially, the newborn receives passive antibodies, mainly immunoglobulin A (IgA), from the mother. These antibodies provide protection against potential pathogens until the newborn's immune system has developed and matured, typically by the age of 3 (Zheng et al., 2020). The early period is critical, as the infant's microbiome must be established properly to support the development of the immune system and maintain homeostasis. The interaction between the infant's microbiota and immune system is essential for the formation of lymphoid structures, immune cells, and functions that safeguard the host against pathogens and tumors. Any disturbances in this process may lead to improper immune system development, increased susceptibility to infections, and other long-lasting effects on the host (Zheng et al., 2020).

The microbiota plays a crucial role in regulating immune responses to pathogens and tumors, which includes effective responses to immunotherapies (Fig. 1). Conversely, the microbiota can also contribute to inflammation, increase susceptibility to infections, and lead to immunosuppression, as well as affect the outcomes and complications of immunotherapies. For these reasons, it is essential to understand the relationship between the microbiome and the host immune system to effectively control and prevent pathogens and tumors (Li et al., 2024; Zhou et al., 2021). Over the past few decades, research including the microbiome has primarily used murine models and patient samples to develop of therapeutic strategies and diagnostic tools (Kandalai et al., 2023). However, most studies have focused on the general population and have limited representation from underrepresented communities, such as AI/AN. Furthermore, AI/AN communities are disproportionately impacted by healthcare and education disparities (Stebbins et al., 2019; White et al., 2014). These disparities can negatively affect AI/AN, highlighting the need to study and understand the increased risk factors that contribute to socioeconomic and ethnic–racial disparities.

3.4 Modulating the Microbiome

In the last decade, studies have revealed a promising strategy for enhancing the effectiveness of immunotherapies and other cancer treatments through microbiome modulation. This approach involves using beneficial microbes, such as probiotics, prebiotics, microbial transplants, and microbial products, to positively influence the microbiota. Such modifications may lead to improved immune responses, better pathogen clearance, enhanced cancer treatments, prevention of diseases, and reduced inflammation in various ways (Huang et al., 2024; Li et al., 2024). However, the methods are relatively new and necessitate further research to understand the specific mechanisms at play, identify the particular microbes involved, and ensure the inclusion of AI/AN populations in clinical studies. We are beginning to gain insight into the microbial composition of the gut, gastric, and vaginal microbiomes within AI/AN communities through the current projects mentioned. Additionally, we are collaborating with community partners, members, and our advisory board to incorporate Indigenous perspectives into our findings and to contextualize our results for sharing with the AI/AN communities involved in these projects (Fig. 2). By integrating various strategies to understand and treat infectious diseases and cancers, we aim to improve health and educational disparities, specifically related to cancer in AI/AN communities (Fig. 1).

3.5 *Restoring Balance*

When considering various approaches to cancer treatment and prevention, it is essential to recognize the available options and their associated risks. Precision medicine can help address some of the challenges in this area. This model customizes treatments to meet the individual needs of patients by utilizing information such as microbiome composition, lifestyle factors, and genetic data. Genetics, in particular, can provide crucial insights for precision medicine by revealing health factors such as blood type, predisposition to certain illnesses, and potential cancer biomarkers (Claw et al., 2024; Jotshi et al., 2023). To effectively interpret and apply these tools for improving healthcare, knowledge, and cancer treatment outcomes, collaboration among experts in fields such as immunology, microbiology, biochemistry, public health, and others is necessary. Personalized interventions in this context require further research and insight from AI/AN communities (Trinidad et al., 2022). Implementing cultural concepts within research methodologies, such as the use of talking circles, is crucial for understanding tribal dynamics and thus potential effective treatment and prevention of diseases and cancers. However, existing barriers, including medical distrust and inadequate access to healthcare, impede the progress of precision medicine (Bordeaux et al., 2021). Building trust with the tribes we work with is vital to our research and ongoing collaboration to treat and prevent cancers among AI/AN populations. We aim to collaborate closely with organizations that educate and provide training on Indigenous data sovereignty and governance, such as the Indigenous DataSET (Institute, 2025). Additionally, we plan to connect with Indigenous-led biorepositories, such as the Native BioData Consortia, to ensure that data is maintained and handled respectfully (Garba et al., 2023). Initiatives such as these and the NACP will continue to implement and uphold the "two-eyed seeing" paradigm (Fig. 2), which can help address health equity for AI/AN populations.

4 Gastric Cancer: Role of *Helicobacter pylori* and Microbiome

Helicobacter pylori (*H. pylori*) is a spiral-shaped, gram-negative bacterium that colonizes the human stomach. It is one of the most prevalent chronic bacterial infections worldwide, affecting over half of the global population, with infection rates ranging from 80% in developing countries to 20–25% among developed countries (McColl, 2010; Zamani et al., 2018). *H. pylori* infection is the leading cause of various gastric diseases, including functional dyspepsia, gastritis, gastroduodenal ulcers, gastric adenocarcinoma, and mucosa-associated lymphoid tissue (MALT) lymphoma (Correa, 1992; Crowe, 2019). *H. pylori* is one of the most common infectious agents linked to any malignancy (de Martel et al., 2012). The relative risk ratio of gastric cancer (GC) associated with *H. pylori* is 5.8 when compared to individuals with healthy stomachs and 9.1 in the presence of atrophic gastritis (Vohlonen et al., 2016). While uncertainty remains regarding the mode of transmission, it is believed to spread from person-to-person through the fecal–oral route (Bui et al., 2016). Acquisition of *H. pylori* infection probably occurs in childhood and can persist into adulthood if untreated (Brown, 2000; McColl, 2010).

While globally, GC remains the fifth leading cause of cancer and the third most deadly, the overall incidence has declined in the U.S. (Makola et al., 2007; Rawla & Barsouk, 2019). Despite global decreasing trends, GC cases and deaths are expected to rise among certain populations (International Agency for Research on Cancer, 2014). Incidence rates of GC among AI/AN are higher than non-Hispanic Whites (NHW) across most of the U.S., with 3.4 times higher rates in the Southwest Indian Health Service region (Brown, 2000; Makola et al., 2007). Among the Navajo population, GC is the sixth highest diagnosed cancer with over 3 times higher incidence compared to Arizona/New Mexico NHW (Melkonian et al., 2020; Weir et al., 2008). Because of its late diagnosis, Navajos are 4.4 times more likely to die from GC compared to NHW (NEC). Furthermore, GC 5-year survival is low among AI/AN males (19.3%) and females (31.1%) (NEC; Weir et al., 2008). The high burden of *H. pylori* infection in AI communities has been attributed to various factors (Fig. 3), including overcrowded living conditions, lack of access to clean water and sanitation, and traditional dietary practices (Driscoll et al., 2017; Miernyk et al., 2018). Our study in Northern Arizona has shown an *H. pylori* prevalence rate of 56% in the Navajo Nation, with 72% of households having at least one infected person (Harris et al., 2022; Pete et al., 2024). A significant risk factor was associated with unregulated water compared with households that used regulated water, and males had 3.3 higher odds of *H. pylori* infection than females (Harris et al., 2022).

H. pylori infection can be treated using diverse antibiotics and proton pump inhibitors (PPI) (Fig. 3) (Malfertheiner et al., 2017; Mannion et al., 2021). The first-line therapy consists of a PPI, amoxicillin plus clarithromycin or metronidazole for 14 days (Chey et al., 2007; Graham & Moss, 2022). If the treatment fails, a second-line therapy is used consisting of a PPI plus tetracycline, metronidazole, and bismuth subcitrate (Ho et al., 2022; Shah et al., 2021). The rate of antimicrobial

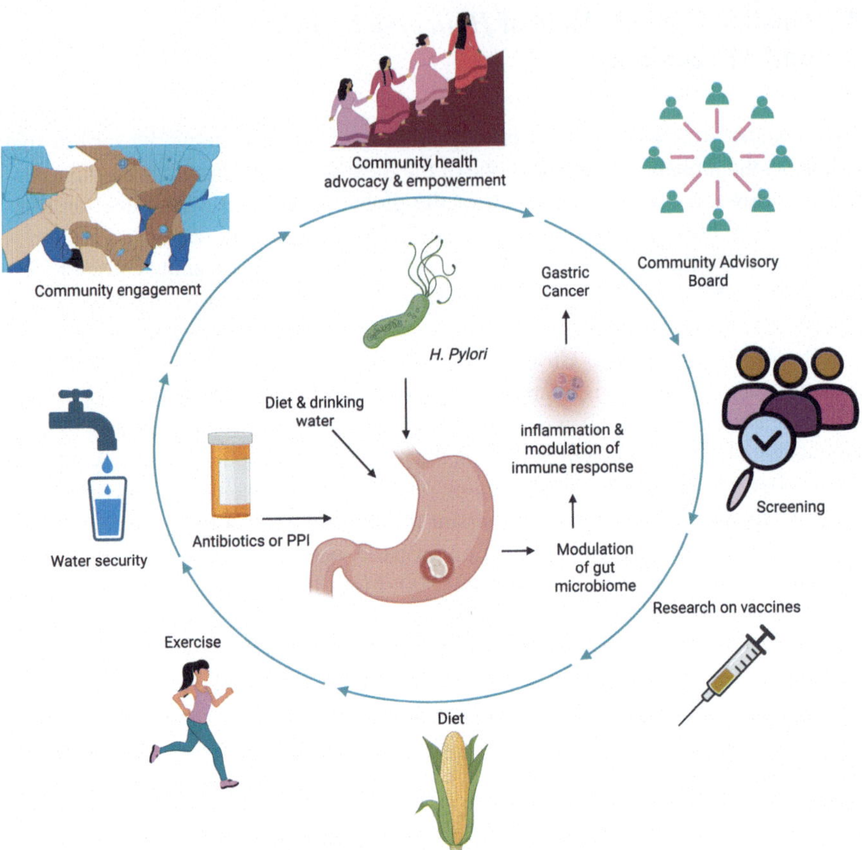

Fig. 3 *H. pylori*, gastric cancer, and prevention. Infection with *H. pylori* in individuals can lead to various health issues that may be worsened by diet, drinking water quality, and the use of antibiotic or PPIs. These factors can influence the gut microbiome and immune response, potentially increasing the risk of gastric cancer. Preventing *H. pylori* infections and gastric cancer involves several strategies, including raising awareness, incorporating AI/AN perspectives, and promoting a positive diet and exercise for healthier lifestyles

resistance in the Navajo Nation is unknown. However, *H. pylori* eradication failure in this population is the result of a combination of factors such as patient compliance, antimicrobial resistance, empirical treatments used by providers across Indian Health Care Centers, lack of provider awareness of local and national resistance patterns for specific antibiotics, and the lack of culture-driven therapy for increased eradication success (Monroy et al., 2023). This has resulted in overuse of antibiotics in the quest to eradicate this infection.

One of the overlooked side effects of antibiotic overuse is its impact on the gastric microbiome, disrupting the microbe–host interactions at the gastric mucosa and potentially exacerbating the progression of *H. pylori* infection and associated inflammatory response. The human microbiome refers to the collection of microorganisms, including bacteria, viruses, fungi, and their genetic material, that reside in and on the human body, playing a critical role in maintaining health and preventing disease. The role of the intestinal microbiome in health and disease has been well studied, but the role of the gastric microbiome is less well-defined. Antibiotic use, even short-term, can have pervasive and lasting effects on the gut microbiome (Jernberg et al., 2010; Ramirez et al., 2020). In the lower intestinal tract, antibiotic therapy can reduce microbial diversity (Palleja et al., 2018), alter metabolic function (Choo et al., 2017), and lead to the persistence of antibiotic-resistant organisms (Ramirez et al., 2020; Xu et al., 2020). Recovery of the gut microbiota after antibiotic treatment is highly dependent on the individual and antibiotic therapy regimen. In a study of healthy adults, a 4-day intervention with meropenem, gentamicin, and vancomycin resulted in an initial overgrowth of pathobionts (e.g., *Enterococcus*) and depletion of *Bifidobacterium* and other beneficial microbes (Palleja et al., 2018). After about 1.5 months, the baseline microbiome mostly recovered, but several taxa that were present at baseline were undetectable after 180 days (Palleja et al., 2018). In the stomach, both PPIs and antibiotics can change the pH and microbial composition (Minalyan et al., 2017; von Rosenvinge et al., 2013). One study demonstrated that the standard of care antibiotic regimen for *H. pylori* infection reduced bacterial, but not fungal, diversity (von Rosenvinge et al., 2013). Long-term PPI usage results in colonization of the gastric mucosa by oral and lower GI-associated microbiota (Sanduleanu et al., 2001). In a small study of 24 patients, PPI use was associated with increased *Streptococcaceae* in the gastric mucosa, regardless of *H. pylori* infection (Paroni Sterbini et al., 2016; Sanduleanu et al., 2001). The authors suggest that *Streptococcus* may be an indicator species for gastric microbiome alterations in dyspeptic patients. Antibiotics and PPIs are critical first- and second-line treatments for *H. pylori* infection. However, appropriate antibiotic stewardship may reduce the short- and long-term impacts on the gastric and intestinal microbiota.

Preventive strategies for *H. pylori* infection and gastric cancer may involve several approaches (Fig. 3). Although there are currently no approved vaccines for *H. pylori*, ongoing research shows promise in eliminating the need for antibiotics, which could help reduce antibiotic resistance and minimize disturbances to the gut microbiome (Yunle et al., 2024). Common screening methods for detecting *H. pylori* include blood tests, stool tests, endoscopy, and carbon urea breath tests (Dore & Pes, 2021). However, some of these tests may be invasive or difficult to access. In a study conducted within the Navajo Nation, the carbon urea breath test has been used as a noninvasive screening method alongside biopsies, indicating its potential for wider application (Monroy et al., 2022). Other preventive measures involve community health advocacy, such as promoting health lifestyles in the community, by providing information on diet and exercise to prevent health issues related to *H. pylori* and gastric cancer.

Our research on the gastric microbiome aligns with the "two-eyed seeing" paradigm (Fig. 2) by integrating Indigenous knowledge with Western biomedical approaches to address the high burden of *H. pylori* infection and gastric cancer among the Navajo population. We recognize the importance of environmental, cultural, and historical factors contributing to disease risk. By incorporating Indigenous perspectives on health, water security, and traditional dietary practices alongside Western medical treatments, we aim for a more holistic approach. Additionally, by exploring the impact of antibiotic overuse on the gastric microbiome, this research recognizes the interconnectedness of healthy central principle in many Indigenous worldviews. Implementing cultural approaches such as education, screening initiatives, and discussions with AI/AN communities is essential for effective cancer prevention and treatment. Collaborating with Indigenous communities fosters a more comprehensive and culturally informed strategy to improve health outcomes and promote sustainable, effective treatment strategies.

5 HPV, Vaginal Microbiome, and Cervical Cancer

Human papillomavirus (HPV) is the most common sexually transmitted infection (STI) in the U.S., with over 200 HPV genotypes that cause an estimated 6.2 million newly infected individuals each year (Weinstock et al., 2004). There are 14 oncogenic or high-risk (hrHPV) genotypes that cause nearly all cervical cancers, a leading malignancy in women globally (Munoz et al., 2003). In the U.S., over 11,500 cases of cervical cancer were diagnosed in 2020, and annual mortality exceeded 4000 (CDC, 2023b). According to Indian Health Service data from 1999 to 2009, Native American women had approximately a two-fold higher incidence and associated mortality rate than White women (White et al., 2014). Between 2016 and 2020, Hispanic and AI/AN women had the highest age-adjusted rates of cervical cancer in Native Americans from Arizona, with 7.8 and 7.1 cases per 100,000 women, compared to 5.6 in NHW women (CDC, 2023b). Innovation in prevention, screening, and care methods are increasing, but Native American and Hispanic women are still disproportionally impacted by cervical cancer. These populations tend to receive diagnosis later and at more advanced stages than NHWs (Holt et al., 2023). Furthermore, this data was supported by differences in late-stage cancers in geographic locations with differences in race/ethnicity, U.S.-born status, and socioeconomic status (Sokale et al., 2023). Due to these differences in diagnosis, it is not surprising that associated mortality rates were also 1.5 times higher in Hispanic women compared to NHW, whereas data on AI/AN were not available (CDC, 2023b). This cervical cancer disparity is attributed to a lack of screening, transportation, medical mistrust, family responsibilities, unequal access and continuity of healthcare, health literacy, and cultural misconceptions and beliefs (Akinlotan et al., 2017; Cesario, 2001; Henderson et al., 2018; Maar et al., 2013; Muslin, 2024; Nugus et al., 2018). In 2021, one in four women were not up to date with their cervical cancer screening, with screening rates lowest among uninsured, recent immigrants, and people without a high school education (ACS, 2024). Other factors, such as a higher prevalence of hrHPV in Native American and Hispanic women are also likely to contribute based on our previous findings (Bell et al., 2011; Leyden et al., 2005).

Globally, the most common hrHPV genotypes are HPV-16, 18, 31, 52, and 58 (Bordeaux et al., 2021; Bruni et al., 2010). In North America, most common types were HPV-16 (5.8%), 18 (2.3%), 52 (2.1%), and 58/51 (combined, 1.5%). Few studies were conducted to estimate hrHPV prevalence within Native American communities. Among those studies, 22.2% of Native American women from the Hopi reservation in Northeastern Arizona tested positive for hrHPV infection (Winer et al., 2016). Recently, we reported on the largest study to estimate hrHPV prevalence among Native American women (Lee et al., 2019). Of the 698 Native American women from a single tribe in the Great Plains, 34.8% were positive for at least one hrHPV (Lee et al., 2019). Most concerning was the elevated hrHPV prevalence among Native American women over 30 years of age, who are at most risk for developing cervical cancer. The deficiencies of both cervical screening and higher HPV prevalence, specifically emerging hrHPV genotypes that are not covered by current or former HPV vaccines (Gholamzad et al., 2024; Lee et al., 2019), are likely contributors to cervical cancer disparities among Native American women. However, further research on the cervicovaginal microenvironment may elucidate other drivers of hrHPV persistence and cancer progression in Indigenous communities (Morales et al., 2022) and identify targets for improved intervention strategies.

Dysbiosis has recently been implicated in the development of cancer, including cervical cancer (Laniewski et al., 2020b; Raskov et al., 2017). In the majority of healthy reproductive-age women, vaginal microbiota is dominated by *Lactobacillus* species (Fig. 4), which are known to protect the host from many urogenital diseases (bacterial vaginosis, yeast infections, and STI) by lowering vaginal pH through lactic acid production and the secretion of antimicrobial compounds (Ravel et al., 2011). Bacterial vaginosis (BV), the most common vaginal disorder of reproductive-age women, is associated with a quantitative decline in lactobacilli numbers, as well as obstetric and gynecologic sequelae, and an increased risk of STI acquisition, including HPV (Marrazzo, 2006). BV-associated organisms include obligate and facultative anaerobic bacteria, such as *Gardnerella vaginalis*, *Fannyhessea vaginae*, *Prevotella bivia*, *Megasphaera*, *Sneathia*, *Peptoniphilus*, *Porphyromonas*, and others; several of which have been identified as key microbes in modulation of a gynecologic cancer microenvironment (Laniewski et al., 2020b). In vitro analysis of *Sneathia*, *Fannyhessea*, and *Peptoniphilus* altered hallmarks of cancer, including robust proinflammatory, oxidative stress-associated compounds and disruption to the epithelial cell barrier (Laniewski & Herbst-Kralovetz, 2021; Maarsingh et al., 2022).

Lactobacillus colonization can be disrupted by many factors, including behavioral factors (smoking, age of sexual debut, sexual activity, use of lubricants and sex toys, contraception, alcohol consumption), clinical factors (hormonal status, contraception, vaccination status, hormonal dysregulation conditions such as obesity), environmental factors (geographic location, stress and trauma, use of drugs, supplements, or antibiotics), and social factors (socioeconomic status, race/ethnicity, education level, access to care) and immunological factors (age, epigenetics, altered immunity, comorbidities) (Fig. 1) (Laniewski et al., 2020b; Morales et al., 2022). More recent research involving the microbiome and societal stress and

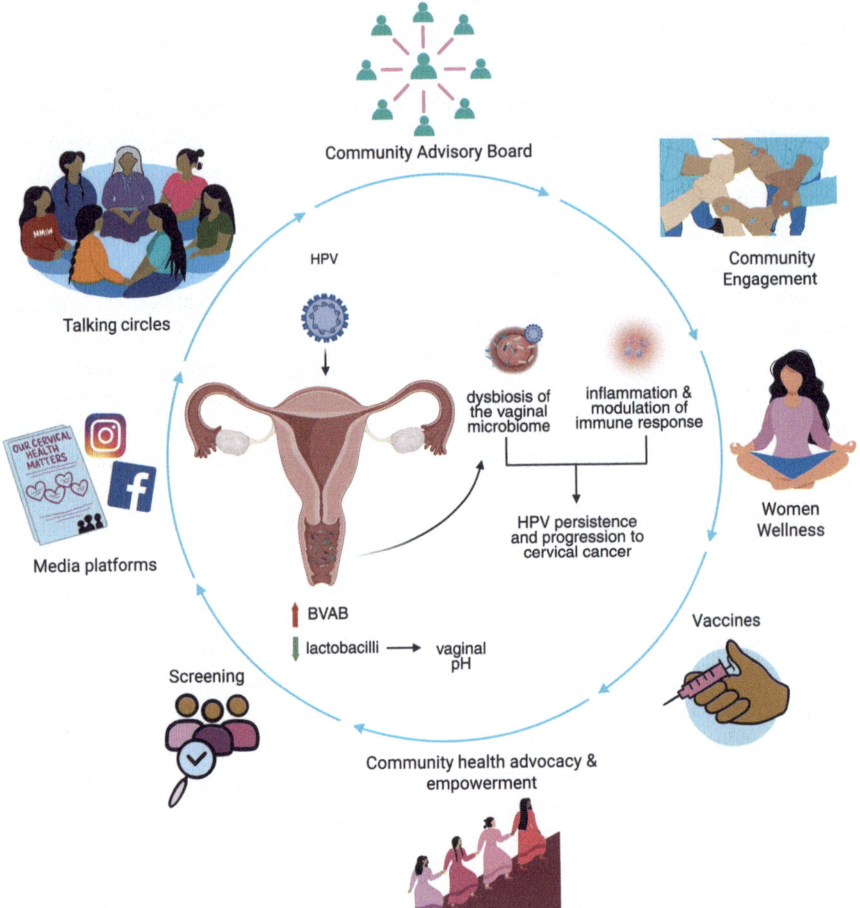

Fig. 4 HPV, cervical cancer, and prevention. Infection with HPV, especially high-risk, is known to affect the vaginal microbiome, potentially leading to an increase in bacterial vaginosis-associated bacteria (BVAB) and a decrease in beneficial microbes such as lactobacilli. This imbalance can alter vaginal pH and immune responses, resulting in HPV persistence and an increased risk of cervical cancer. Understanding the factors that contribute to cervical cancer among AI/AN populations and sharing this knowledge is crucial in addressing HPV infections and reducing cancer risk. This project outlines several strategies to prevent HPV and cervical cancer, including talking circles, vaccination, promoting women's wellness, and advocating for community health

discrimination (Beurel, 2024; Dong et al., 2024; Rawson, 2024) are areas of interest that may further shed light on the role of the microbiome in health disparities related to HPV infection and cervical cancer.

Notably, HPV-infected women exhibit a more diverse vaginal microbiome and lower *Lactobacillus* levels relative to healthy HPV-negative women (Gao et al., 2013; Laniewski et al., 2020b; Mitra et al., 2016). Although persistent HPV infection is the primary cause of precancerous cervical intraepithelial neoplasia and invasive cervical carcinoma (Ho et al., 1995), only a small portion of women infected with HPV progress to dysplasia and, if not treated, to cancer (Shulzhenko et al., 2014). Numerous cross-sectional studies illuminated associations between vaginal microbiota composition, HPV persistence, and cervical cancer progression (Audirac-Chalifour et al., 2016; Carter et al., 2021; Cheng et al., 2020; Godoy-Vitorino et al., 2018; Kwasniewski et al., 2018; Laniewski et al., 2018; Lee et al., 2013; Oh et al., 2015; Onywera et al., 2019; Piyathilake et al., 2016); however, studies with a longitudinal design or inclusion of diverse populations disproportionally affected by disease are still limited (Brotman et al., 2014; Di Paola et al., 2017; Mei et al., 2022; Mitra et al., 2015; Shannon et al., 2017; Usyk et al., 2020). A 2019 study also demonstrated an association between HPV infection, cervical carcinogenesis, and the diverse vaginal microbiota (VMB) in a cohort of Hispanic and non-Hispanic women from the Phoenix, Arizona, metropolitan area. Through multi-omics approaches (Bokulich et al., 2022), we identified microbial (e.g., *Sneathia*, *Atopobiaceae*, and increased species diversity) (Jimenez et al., 2024; Laniewski et al., 2018), metabolic (Ilhan et al., 2019), and immune signatures associated with cervical carcinogenesis (Laniewski et al., 2019; Laniewski et al., 2020a). Furthermore, a 2018 meta-analysis of longitudinal studies, conducted mostly in European and NHW populations, supported a causal link between a diverse *Lactobacillus*-depleted microbiome and HPV acquisition, HPV persistence, and development of cervical dysplasia (Brusselaers et al., 2019). Another meta-analysis also revealed that women with diverse VMB dominated by anaerobic bacteria or *Lactobacillus iners* had higher odds of high-risk HPV prevalence and cervical dysplasia compared to women with microbiota dominated by *Lactobacillus crispatus* (Norenhag et al., 2020; Wang et al., 2019). Further, a systematic review on studies conducted in North and South America among Latina populations identified seven enriched species including *Sneathia*, *Chlamydia*, and *Prevotella* with HPV infection, cervical dysplasia, or cervical cancer (Mancilla et al., 2024).

Despite differences in cervical cancer rates between racial and ethnic groups, little is known about the patterns of HPV infection, the composition of the vaginal microbiota in Native American communities, or how these factors relate to increased cervical cancer risk. In fact, most prior studies do not include Native American women. In our pilot study funded by the National Cancer Institute (NCI) through NACP, 31 participants were recruited in 2019–2021 at the Native Americans Community Action (NACA) clinic in Flagstaff, AZ (Laniewski et al., 2024). HrHPV genotypes (HPV-39, 45, 52, 53, 58, 59) were detected in 23% of women (five Native American and two non-Native). Notably, the current nonavalent HPV vaccine does not target half of the genotypes detected in this cohort. Vaginal microbiota profiles were dominated by *Lactobacillus* in 44% of Native American women, compared to 58% in non-Native participants, which is overall lower than in previously reported NHW cohorts. The most prevalent *Lactobacillus* species included *L. crispatus* (associated with optimal health) and *L. iners* (considered nonoptimal) (Petrova et al., 2017). *Lactobacillus*-depleted profiles consisted of typical communities of BV-associated anaerobes: *Gardnerella*, *Fannyhessea*, *Prevotella*, and *Sneathia* (Muzny et al., 2020). *Lactobacillus* dominance was highly associated with acidic vaginal pH. Intriguingly, the vaginal microbiota of Native American women was highly enriched in *Sneathia* (previously identified to be also enriched in Hispanic women). Moreover, HPV-positive individuals tended to have lower *Lactobacillus* abundance compared to HPV-negative women. Immune marker profiles also related to the vaginal microbiota composition with proinflammatory cytokines being elevated in women with *Lactobacillus* depletion. We also evaluated *Lactobacillus* dominance within the vaginal microbiome in the context of sociodemographic and lifestyle factors. We observed associations of multiple people in a household, lower level of education, and high parity to undesirable non-*Lactobacillus*-dominant microbiota and abundance of specific bacterial species. Thus, these factors might contribute to cervical carcinogenesis via alteration of vaginal microbiota. Overall, our pilot study suggests that an interplay between HPV, vaginal microbiome and host defense may play a role in cervical cancer health disparity among Native American women. This study also provided the foundation for ongoing and future longitudinal studies required to better understand the mechanistic role of vaginal microbiota in HPV persistence or HPV clearance and the contribution of social determinants of health in cervical cancer health disparities among AI/AN population.

Our ongoing research includes basic science, translational cancer prevention, and training components that align with the goals of the overall NACP project. We utilize the "two-eyed seeing" paradigm (Fig. 2) in our study. We currently collaborate with a significant community partner, the MedStar Health Research Institute in Phoenix, AZ, which has a long history of serving urban Native populations in Arizona. This partnership with MedStar is essential to our research, enabling us to build relationships with tribes through activities such as talking circles, survey collection, noninvasive biological specimen collection, community engagement, and overall community building (Fig. 4). Recently, we implemented talking circles to gather community perspectives on our research and identify effective methods for disseminating new information in a culturally appropriate manner to the urban Native communities involved in the research. Additionally, our team regularly communicates and updates the development of culturally informed data collection protocols and surveys. We are utilizing various educational materials, including text messages, social media posts, websites, flyers, and pamphlets, to inform communities about HPV and cervical cancer prevention, as well as to promote women's wellness exams. These exams are crucial for addressing both reproductive and overall health, including early detection of abnormal cervical cells and contributing to well-being and restoring balance. Our ongoing efforts focus on expanding and developing strategies for treatment, prevention, and in-person education. We aim to establish educational tools that empower tribes to advocate for the health of their communities. While HPV vaccination and annual Well women's exams are the primary forms of cervical cancer prevention and detection, through collaboration with our partners and the community, we are working to address this public health crisis by incorporating Native American voices and cultural beliefs, which are vital to the prevention and elimination of cervical cancer in Indigenous populations (Whop et al., 2021).

6 Conclusion

Since the beginning of the Human Microbiome Project, trillions of microbes that make up the human microbiome have been identified (Lloyd-Price et al., 2016). However, as Indigenous people, we have embraced importance of balance and harmony within oneself, with others and the surroundings. Thus, as researchers and health providers, we understand the complex roles microbes play in health and disease. While both the microbiome and immune responses to tumors have been extensively studied in the general population, there is still a significant gap in understanding how the microbiome affects cancers, immune status, and treatment outcomes in AI/AN populations. Given that AI/AN communities are disproportionately affected by various health issues, including cancer, it is crucial to assess the composition of the microbiome, immune responses, regulation, modulation, and the interplay involved in cancer progression and treatment (Bordeaux et al., 2021). Currently, several therapies are available for cancer patients; however, the type, stage, and location of cancers present different challenges. Gaining insights into the tumor microenvironment and the associated microbiota may help address these challenges and lead to innovative therapies, including personalized medicine aimed at improving cancer outcomes for AI/AN communities. Furthermore, there is a notable lack of research focused on cancer treatments and cancer-specific immune responses within AI/AN populations. Here, we identified potential strategies to address the future of AI/AN cancer research and how these approaches may advance the healthcare of AI/AN and other underrepresented populations.

Acknowledgments We would like to acknowledge Amber Kelly for assisting in the design of the images within the chapter. We are grateful for the Indigenous communities the partnership for Native American Cancer Prevention (NACP) has collaborated over the years. Particularly, we want to acknowledge the staff and healthcare providers at the Native Americans for Community Action (NACA) clinic located in Flagstaff, AZ. We also like to acknowledge MedStar Health Research Industries and the Strong Heart Study team in Phoenix, AZ, as well as the invaluable cooperation of the Navajo Healthy Stomach Project. Finally, we are immensely grateful for NACP Community Advisory Board (CAB) for providing their insight into the chapters message for our communities, healthcare providers, and researchers. Funding: National Cancer Institute (NCI) Comprehensive Partnerships to Advance Cancer Health Equity (CPACHE) (UACC) U54CA143924 and (NAU) U54CA143925.

References

ACS. (2024). *Cancer facts & figures 2024*. American Cancer Society. https://www.cancer.org/research/cancer-facts-statistics/all-cancer-facts-figures/2024-cancer-facts-figures.html

Akinlotan, M., Bolin, J. N., Helduser, J., Ojinnaka, C., Lichorad, A., & McClellan, D. (2017). Cervical cancer screening barriers and risk factor knowledge among uninsured women. *Journal of Community Health, 42*(4), 770–778. https://doi.org/10.1007/s10900-017-0316-9

Amir, M., Brown, J. A., Rager, S. L., Sanidad, K. Z., Ananthanarayanan, A., & Zeng, M. Y. (2020). Maternal microbiome and infections in pregnancy. *Microorganisms, 8*(12). https://doi.org/10.3390/microorganisms8121996

Audirac-Chalifour, A., Torres-Poveda, K., Bahena-Roman, M., Tellez-Sosa, J., Martinez-Barnetche, J., Cortina-Ceballos, B., et al. (2016). Cervical microbiome and cytokine profile at various stages of cervical cancer: A pilot study. *PLoS One, 11*(4), e0153274. https://doi.org/10.1371/journal.pone.0153274

Bell, M. C., Schmidt-Grimminger, D., Jacobsen, C., Chauhan, S. C., Maher, D. M., & Buchwald, D. S. (2011). Risk factors for HPV infection among American Indian and white women in the Northern Plains. *Gynecologic Oncology, 121*(3), 532–536. https://doi.org/10.1016/j.ygyno.2011.02.032

Beurel, E. (2024). Stress in the microbiome-immune crosstalk. *Gut Microbes, 16*(1), 2327409. https://doi.org/10.1080/19490976.2024.2327409

Bokulich, N. A., Laniewski, P., Adamov, A., Chase, D. M., Caporaso, J. G., & Herbst-Kralovetz, M. M. (2022). Multi-omics data integration reveals metabolome as the top predictor of the cervicovaginal microenvironment. *PLoS Computational Biology, 18*(2), e1009876. https://doi.org/10.1371/journal.pcbi.1009876

Bordeaux, S. J., Baca, A. W., Begay, R. L., Gachupin, F. C., Caporaso, J. G., Herbst-Kralovetz, M. M., & Lee, N. R. (2021). Designing inclusive HPV cancer vaccines and increasing uptake among Native Americans-A cultural perspective review. *Current Oncology, 28*(5), 3705–3716. https://doi.org/10.3390/curroncol28050316

Brotman, R. M., Shardell, M. D., Gajer, P., Tracy, J. K., Zenilman, J. M., Ravel, J., & Gravitt, P. E. (2014). Interplay between the temporal dynamics of the vaginal microbiota and human papillomavirus detection. *The Journal of Infectious Diseases, 210*(11), 1723–1733. https://doi.org/10.1093/infdis/jiu330

Brown, L. M. (2000). Helicobacter pylori: Epidemiology and routes of transmission. *Epidemiologic Reviews, 22*(2), 283–297. https://doi.org/10.1093/oxfordjournals.epirev.a018040

Bruni, L., Diaz, M., Castellsagué, X., Ferrer, E., Bosch, F. X., & de Sanjosé, S. (2010). Cervical human papillomavirus prevalence in 5 continents: Meta-analysis of 1 million women with normal cytological findings. *The Journal of Infectious Diseases, 202*(12), 1789–1799. https://doi.org/10.1086/657321

Brusselaers, N., Shrestha, S., van de Wijgert, J., & Verstraelen, H. (2019). Vaginal dysbiosis and the risk of human papillomavirus and cervical cancer: Systematic review and meta-analysis. *American Journal of Obstetrics and Gynecology, 221*(1), 9–18 e18. https://doi.org/10.1016/j.ajog.2018.12.011

Bui, D., Brown, H. E., Harris, R. B., & Oren, E. (2016). Serologic evidence for fecal-oral transmission of Helicobacter pylori. *The American Journal of Tropical Medicine and Hygiene, 94*(1), 82–88. https://doi.org/10.4269/ajtmh.15-0297

Burhansstipanov, L., Braun, K. L., Blanchard, J., Petereit, D., Olson, A. K., Sanderson, P. R., et al. (2022). Cancer and survivorship in American Indians and Alaska Natives. In *Indigenous public health* (pp. 147–173). University Press of Kentucky. https://doi.org/10.5810/kentucky/9780813195841.001.0001

Carter, K. A., Srinivasan, S., Fiedler, T. L., Anzala, O., Kimani, J., Mochache, V., et al. (2021). Vaginal bacteria and risk of incident and persistent infection with high-risk subtypes of human papillomavirus: A cohort study among Kenyan women. *Sexually Transmitted Diseases, 48*(7), 499–507. https://doi.org/10.1097/OLQ.0000000000001343

CDC. (2023a). *Health, United States, annual perspective 2020–2021*. NCHS Health, United States, Issue. https://stacks.cdc.gov/view/cdc/122044

CDC. (2023b). *United States cancer statistics: Data visualizations*. https://www.cdc.gov/cancer/uscs/dataviz/index.htm

Cesario, S. K. (2001). Care of the Native American woman: Strategies for practice, education, and research. *Journal of Obstetric, Gynecologic, and Neonatal Nursing, 30*(1), 13–19.

Cheng, L., Norenhag, J., Hu, Y. O. O., Brusselaers, N., Fransson, E., Ahrlund-Richter, A., et al. (2020). Vaginal microbiota and human papillomavirus infection among young Swedish women. *NPJ Biofilms and Microbiomes, 6*(1), 39. https://doi.org/10.1038/s41522-020-00146-8

Chey, W. D., Wong, B. C., & Practice Parameters Committee of the American College of Gastroenterology. (2007). American College of Gastroenterology guideline on the management of Helicobacter pylori infection. *The American Journal of Gastroenterology, 102*(8), 1808–1825. https://doi.org/10.1111/j.1572-0241.2007.01393.x

Choo, J. M., Kanno, T., Zain, N. M., Leong, L. E., Abell, G. C., Keeble, J. E., et al. (2017). Divergent relationships between fecal microbiota and metabolomc following distinct antibiotic-induced disruptions. *mSphere, 2*(1). https://doi.org/10.1128/mSphere.00005-17

Claw, G. K., Dorr, R. C., & Woodahl, L. E. (2024). Implementing community-engaged pharmacogenomics in Indigenous communities. *Nature Communications, 15*(1). https://doi.org/10.1038/s41467-024-45032-5

Correa, P. (1992). Human gastric carcinogenesis: a multistep and multifactorial process–First American Cancer Society Award Lecture on Cancer Epidemiology and Prevention. *Cancer Research, 52*(24), 6735–6740.

Crowe, S. E. (2019). Helicobacter pylori infection. *The New England Journal of Medicine, 380*(12), 1158–1165. https://doi.org/10.1056/NEJMcp1710945

de Martel, C., Ferlay, J., Franceschi, S., Vignat, J., Bray, F., Forman, D., & Plummer, M. (2012). Global burden of cancers attributable to infections in 2008: A review and synthetic analysis. *The Lancet Oncology, 13*(6), 607–615. https://doi.org/10.1016/S1470-2045(12)70137-7

Di Paola, M., Sani, C., Clemente, A. M., Iossa, A., Perissi, E., Castronovo, G., et al. (2017). Characterization of cervico-vaginal microbiota in women developing persistent high-risk Human Papillomavirus infection. *Scientific Reports, 7*(1), 10200. https://doi.org/10.1038/s41598-017-09842-6

Dong, T. S., Shera, S., Peters, K., Gee, G. C., Beltran-Sanchez, H., Wang, M. C., et al. (2024). Experiences of discrimination are associated with microbiome and transcriptome alterations in the gut. *Frontiers in Microbiology, 15*, 1457028. https://doi.org/10.3389/fmicb.2024.1457028

Dore, P. M., & Pes, M. G. (2021). What is new in Helicobacter pylori diagnosis. An Overview. *Journal of Clinical Medicine, 10*(10), 2091. https://doi.org/10.3390/jcm10102091

Driscoll, L. J., Brown, H. E., Harris, R. B., & Oren, E. (2017). Population knowledge, attitude, and practice regarding Helicobacter pylori transmission and outcomes: A literature review. *Frontiers in Public Health, 5*, 144. https://doi.org/10.3389/fpubh.2017.00144

Du, S., Yan, J., Xue, Y., Zhong, Y., & Dong, Y. (2023). Adoptive cell therapy for cancer treatment. *Exploration (Beijing), 3*(4), 20210058. https://doi.org/10.1002/EXP.20210058

Emole, J., Lawal, O., Lupak, O., Dias, A., Shune, L., & Yusuf, K. (2022). Demographic differences among patients treated with chimeric antigen receptor T-cell therapy in the United States. *Cancer Medicine, 11*(23), 4440–4448. https://doi.org/10.1002/cam4.4797

Feng, Q., Sun, B., Xue, T., Li, R., Lin, C., Gao, Y., et al. (2022). Advances in CAR T-cell therapy in bile duct, pancreatic, and gastric cancers. *Frontiers in Immunology, 13*, 1025608. https://doi.org/10.3389/fimmu.2022.1025608

Gachupin, F. C., Ingram, J. C., Laurila, K. A., Lluria-Prevatt, M. C., Teufel-Shone, N. I., & Briehl, M. M. (2021). NACP: Partnership for Native American cancer prevention. *Cancer Health Disparities, 5*, 164.

Gao, W., Weng, J., Gao, Y., & Chen, X. (2013). Comparison of the vaginal microbiota diversity of women with and without human papillomavirus infection: A cross-sectional study. *BMC Infectious Diseases, 13*, 271. https://doi.org/10.1186/1471-2334-13-271

Garba, I., Sterling, R., Plevel, R., Carson, W., Cordova-Marks, M. F., Cummins, J., et al. (2023). Indigenous peoples and research: Self-determination in research governance. *Frontiers in Research Metrics and Analytics, 8*. https://doi.org/10.3389/frma.2023.1272318

Gholamzad, A., Khakpour, N., Hashemi, M., & Gholamzad, M. (2024). Prevalence of high and low risk HPV genotypes among vaccinated and non-vaccinated people in Tehran. *Virology Journal, 21*(1), 9. https://doi.org/10.1186/s12985-023-02270-1

Godoy-Vitorino, F., Romaguera, J., Zhao, C., Vargas-Robles, D., Ortiz-Morales, G., Vazquez-Sanchez, F., et al. (2018). Cervicovaginal fungi and bacteria associated with cervical intraepithelial neoplasia and high-risk human papillomavirus infections in a Hispanic population. *Frontiers in Microbiology, 9*, 2533. https://doi.org/10.3389/fmicb.2018.02533

Graham, D. Y., & Moss, S. F. (2022). Antimicrobial susceptibility testing for Helicobacter pylori is now widely available: When, how, why. *The American Journal of Gastroenterology, 117*(4), 524–528. https://doi.org/10.14309/ajg.0000000000001659

Guadagnolo, B. A., Petereit, D. G., & Coleman, C. N. (2017). Cancer care access and outcomes for American Indian populations in the United States: Challenges and models for progress. *Seminars in Radiation Oncology, 27*(2), 143–149. https://doi.org/10.1016/j.semradonc.2016.11.006

Harris, R. B., Brown, H. E., Begay, R. L., Sanderson, P. R., Chief, C., Monroy, F. P., & Oren, E. (2022). Helicobacter pylori prevalence and risk factors in three rural indigenous communities of northern Arizona. *International Journal of Environmental Research and Public Health, 19*(2). https://doi.org/10.3390/ijerph19020797

He, X., & Xu, C. (2020). Immune checkpoint signaling and cancer immunotherapy. *Cell Research, 30*(8), 660–669. https://doi.org/10.1038/s41422-020-0343-4

Hellmann, M. D., Rizvi, N. A., Goldman, J. W., Gettinger, S. N., Borghaei, H., Brahmer, J. R., et al. (2017). Nivolumab plus ipilimumab as first-line treatment for advanced non-small-cell lung cancer (CheckMate 012): Results of an open-label, phase 1, multicohort study. *The Lancet Oncology, 18*(1), 31–41. https://doi.org/10.1016/S1470-2045(16)30624-6

Henderson, R. I., Shea-Budgell, M., Healy, C., Letendre, A., Bill, L., Healy, B., et al. (2018). First nations people's perspectives on barriers and supports for enhancing HPV vaccination: Foundations for sustainable, community-driven strategies. *Gynecologic Oncology, 149*(1), 93–100. https://doi.org/10.1016/j.ygyno.2017.12.024

Ho, G. Y., Burk, R. D., Klein, S., Kadish, A. S., Chang, C. J., Palan, P., et al. (1995). Persistent genital human papillomavirus infection as a risk factor for persistent cervical dysplasia. *Journal of the National Cancer Institute, 87*(18), 1365–1371. https://doi.org/10.1093/jnci/87.18.1365

Ho, J. J. C., Navarro, M., Sawyer, K., Elfanagely, Y., & Moss, S. F. (2022). Helicobacter pylori antibiotic resistance in the United States between 2011 and 2021: A systematic review and meta-analysis. *The American Journal of Gastroenterology, 117*(8), 1221–1230. https://doi.org/10.14309/ajg.0000000000001828

Holt, H. K., Peterson, C. E., MacLaughlan David, S., Abdelaziz, A., Sawaya, G. F., Guadamuz, J. S., & Calip, G. S. (2023). Mediation of racial and ethnic inequities in the diagnosis of advanced-stage cervical cancer by insurance status. *JAMA Network Open, 6*(3), e232985. https://doi.org/10.1001/jamanetworkopen.2023.2985

Huang, B., Fettweis, J. M., Brooks, J. P., Jefferson, K. K., & Buck, G. A. (2014). The changing landscape of the vaginal microbiome. *Clinics in Laboratory Medicine, 34*(4), 747–761. https://doi.org/10.1016/j.cll.2014.08.006

Huang, R., Liu, Z., Sun, T., & Zhu, L. (2024). Cervicovaginal microbiome, high-risk HPV infection and cervical cancer: Mechanisms and therapeutic potential. *Microbiological Research, 287*, 127857. https://doi.org/10.1016/j.micres.2024.127857

Ilhan, Z. E., Laniewski, P., Thomas, N., Roe, D. J., Chase, D. M., & Herbst-Kralovetz, M. M. (2019). Deciphering the complex interplay between microbiota, HPV, inflammation and cancer through cervicovaginal metabolic profiling. *EBioMedicine, 44*, 675–690. https://doi.org/10.1016/j.ebiom.2019.04.028

Institute, U. o. A. N. N. (2025). *Indigenous DataSET sovereignty & ethics training*. https://nni.arizona.edu/indigenous-dataset

International Agency for Research on Cancer, W. H. O. (2014). *World cancer report 2014*. IARC.

Jernberg, C., Lofmark, S., Edlund, C., & Jansson, J. K. (2010). Long-term impacts of antibiotic exposure on the human intestinal microbiota. *Microbiology (Reading), 156*(Pt 11), 3216–3223. https://doi.org/10.1099/mic.0.040618-0

Jimenez, N. R., Mancilla, V., Laniewski, P., & Herbst-Kralovetz, M. M. (2024). Immunometabolic contributions of Atopobiaceae family members in human papillomavirus infection, cervical dysplasia and cancer. *The Journal of Infectious Diseases*. https://doi.org/10.1093/infdis/jiae533

Jotshi, A., Sukla, K. K., Haque, M. M., Bose, C., Varma, B., Koppiker, C. B., et al. (2023). Exploring the human microbiome – A step forward for precision medicine in breast cancer. *Cancer Reports (Hoboken, N.J.), 6*(11), e1877. https://doi.org/10.1002/cnr2.1877

June, C. H. (2007). Adoptive T cell therapy for cancer in the clinic. *The Journal of Clinical Investigation, 117*(6), 1466–1476. https://doi.org/10.1172/JCI32446

Kahn-John Diné, M., & Koithan, M. (2015). Living in health, harmony, and beauty: The Diné (Navajo) Hózhó wellness philosophy. *Global Advances in Health and Medicine, 4*(3), 24–30. https://doi.org/10.7453/gahmj.2015.044

Kandalai, S., Li, H., Zhang, N., Peng, H., & Zheng, Q. (2023). The human microbiome and cancer: A diagnostic and therapeutic perspective. *Cancer Biology & Therapy, 24*(1), 2240084. https://doi.org/10.1080/15384047.2023.2240084

Kwasniewski, W., Wolun-Cholewa, M., Kotarski, J., Warchol, W., Kuzma, D., Kwasniewska, A., & Gozdzicka-Jozefiak, A. (2018). Microbiota dysbiosis is associated with HPV-induced cervical carcinogenesis. *Oncology Letters, 16*(6), 7035–7047. https://doi.org/10.3892/ol.2018.9509

Laniewski, P., & Herbst-Kralovetz, M. M. (2021). Bacterial vaginosis and health-associated bacteria modulate the immunometabolic landscape in 3D model of human cervix. *NPJ Biofilms and Microbiomes, 7*(1), 88. https://doi.org/10.1038/s41522-021-00259-8

Laniewski, P., Barnes, D., Goulder, A., Cui, H., Roe, D. J., Chase, D. M., & Herbst-Kralovetz, M. M. (2018). Linking cervicovaginal immune signatures, HPV and microbiota composition in cervical carcinogenesis in non-Hispanic and Hispanic women. *Scientific Reports, 8*(1), 7593. https://doi.org/10.1038/s41598-018-25879-7

Laniewski, P., Cui, H., Roe, D. J., Barnes, D., Goulder, A., Monk, B. J., et al. (2019). Features of the cervicovaginal microenvironment drive cancer biomarker signatures in patients across cervical carcinogenesis. *Scientific Reports, 9*(1), 7333. https://doi.org/10.1038/s41598-019-43849-5

Laniewski, P., Cui, H., Roe, D. J., Chase, D. M., & Herbst-Kralovetz, M. M. (2020a). Vaginal microbiota, genital inflammation, and neoplasia impact immune checkpoint protein profiles in the cervicovaginal microenvironment. *NPJ Precision Oncology, 4*, 22. https://doi.org/10.1038/s41698-020-0126-x

Laniewski, P., Ilhan, Z. E., & Herbst-Kralovetz, M. M. (2020b). The microbiome and gynaecological cancer development, prevention and therapy. *Nature Reviews Urology, 17*(4), 232–250. https://doi.org/10.1038/s41585-020-0286-z

Laniewski, P., Joe, T. R., Jimenez, N. R., Eddie, T. L., Bordeaux, S. J., Quiroz, V., et al. (2024). Viewing native American cervical cancer disparities through the lens of the vaginal microbiome: A pilot study. *Cancer Prevention Research, 17*(11), 525–538. https://doi.org/10.1158/1940-6207.CAPR-24-0286

Lee, J. E., Lee, S., Lee, H., Song, Y. M., Lee, K., Han, M. J., et al. (2013). Association of the vaginal microbiota with human papillomavirus infection in a Korean twin cohort. *PLoS One, 8*(5), e63514. https://doi.org/10.1371/journal.pone.0063514

Lee, N. R., Winer, R. L., Cherne, S., Noonan, C. J., Nelson, L., Gonzales, A. A., et al. (2019). Human papillomavirus prevalence among American Indian women of the Great Plains. *The Journal of Infectious Diseases, 219*(6), 908–915. https://doi.org/10.1093/infdis/jiy600

Leyden, W. A., Manos, M. M., Geiger, A. M., Weinmann, S., Mouchawar, J., Bischoff, K., et al. (2005). Cervical cancer in women with comprehensive health care access: Attributable factors in the screening process. *Journal of the National Cancer Institute, 97*(9), 675–683. https://doi.org/10.1093/jnci/dji115

Li, Q., Lei, X., Zhu, J., Zhong, Y., Yang, J., Wang, J., & Tan, H. (2023). Radiotherapy/chemotherapy-immunotherapy for cancer management: From mechanisms to clinical implications. *Oxidative Medicine and Cellular Longevity, 2023*, 7530794. https://doi.org/10.1155/2023/7530794

Li, Z., Xiong, W., Liang, Z., Wang, J., Zeng, Z., Kolat, D., et al. (2024). Critical role of the gut microbiota in immune responses and cancer immunotherapy. *Journal of Hematology & Oncology, 17*(1), 33. https://doi.org/10.1186/s13045-024-01541-w

Lim, K. W. L. (2025). Linking microbiome to cancer: A mini-review on contemporary advances. *The Microbe, 6*, 100279. https://doi.org/10.1016/j.microb.2025.100279

Lin, M. J., Svensson-Arvelund, J., Lubitz, G. S., Marabelle, A., Melero, I., Brown, B. D., & Brody, J. D. (2022). Cancer vaccines: The next immunotherapy frontier. *Nature Cancer, 3*(8), 911–926. https://doi.org/10.1038/s43018-022-00418-6

Liu, Y. P., Zheng, C. C., Huang, Y. N., He, M. L., Xu, W. W., & Li, B. (2021). Molecular mechanisms of chemo- and radiotherapy resistance and the potential implications for cancer treatment. *MedComm (2020), 2*(3), 315–340. https://doi.org/10.1002/mco2.55

Lloyd-Price, J., Abu-Ali, G., & Huttenhower, C. (2016). The healthy human microbiome. *Genome Medicine, 8*(1), 51. https://doi.org/10.1186/s13073-016-0307-y

Lv, B., Wang, Y., Ma, D., Cheng, W., Liu, J., Yong, T., et al. (2022). Immunotherapy: Reshape the tumor immune microenvironment. *Frontiers in Immunology, 13*, 844142. https://doi.org/10.3389/fimmu.2022.844142

Lythgoe, P. M., Mullish, H. B., Frampton, E. A., & Krell, J. (2022). Polymorphic microbes: A new emerging hallmark of cancer. *Trends in Microbiology, 30*(12), 1131–1134. https://doi.org/10.1016/j.tim.2022.08.004

Maar, M., Burchell, A., Little, J., Ogilvie, G., Severini, A., Yang, J. M., & Zehbe, I. (2013). A qualitative study of provider perspectives of structural barriers to cervical cancer screening among first nations women. *Womens Health Issues, 23*(5), e319–e325. https://doi.org/10.1016/j.whi.2013.06.005

Maarsingh, J. D., Laniewski, P., & Herbst-Kralovetz, M. M. (2022). Immunometabolic and potential tumor-promoting changes in 3D cervical cell models infected with bacterial vaginosis-associated bacteria. *Communications Biology, 5*(1), 725. https://doi.org/10.1038/s42003-022-03681-6

Makola, D., Peura, D. A., & Crowe, S. E. (2007). Helicobacter pylori infection and related gastrointestinal diseases. *Journal of Clinical Gastroenterology, 41*(6), 548–558. https://doi.org/10.1097/MCG.0b013e318030e3c3

Malfertheiner, P., Megraud, F., O'Morain, C. A., Gisbert, J. P., Kuipers, E. J., Axon, A. T., et al. (2017). Management of Helicobacter pylori infection-the Maastricht V/Florence consensus report. *Gut, 66*(1), 6–30. https://doi.org/10.1136/gutjnl-2016-312288

Mancilla, V., Jimenez, N. R., Bishop, N. S., Flores, M., & Herbst-Kralovetz, M. M. (2024). The vaginal microbiota, human papillomavirus infection, and cervical carcinogenesis: A systematic review in the Latina population. *Journal of Epidemiology and Global Health, 14*(2), 480–497. https://doi.org/10.1007/s44197-024-00201-z

Mannion, A., Dzink-Fox, J., Shen, Z., Piazuelo, M. B., Wilson, K. T., Correa, P., et al. (2021). Helicobacter pylori antimicrobial resistance and gene variants in high- and low-gastric-cancer-risk populations. *Journal of Clinical Microbiology, 59*(5). https://doi.org/10.1128/JCM.03203-20

Marrazzo, J. M. (2006). A persistent(ly) enigmatic ecological mystery: Bacterial vaginosis. *The Journal of Infectious Diseases, 193*(11), 1475–1477. https://doi.org/10.1086/503783

Martin, D. H. (2012). Two-eyed seeing: A framework for understanding indigenous and non-indigenous approaches to indigenous health research. *The Canadian Journal of Nursing Research, 44*(2), 20–42.

McColl, K. E. (2010). Clinical practice. Helicobacter pylori infection. *The New England Journal of Medicine, 362*(17), 1597–1604. https://doi.org/10.1056/NEJMcp1001110

Mei, L., Wang, T., Chen, Y., Wei, D., Zhang, Y., Cui, T., et al. (2022). Dysbiosis of vaginal microbiota associated with persistent high-risk human papilloma virus infection. *Journal of Translational Medicine, 20*(1), 12. https://doi.org/10.1186/s12967-021-03201-w

Melkonian, S. C., Pete, D., Jim, M. A., Haverkamp, D., Wiggins, C. L., Bruce, M. G., & White, M. C. (2020). Gastric cancer among American Indian and Alaska native populations in the United States, 2005–2016. *The American Journal of Gastroenterology, 115*(12), 1989–1997. https://doi.org/10.14309/ajg.0000000000000748

Miernyk, K. M., Bulkow, L. R., Gold, B. D., Bruce, M. G., Hurlburt, D. H., Griffin, P. M., et al. (2018). Prevalence of Helicobacter pylori among Alaskans: Factors associated with infection and comparison of urea breath test and anti-Helicobacter pylori IgG antibodies. *Helicobacter, 23*(3), e12482. https://doi.org/10.1111/hel.12482

Minalyan, A., Gabrielyan, L., Scott, D., Jacobs, J., & Pisegna, J. R. (2017). The gastric and intestinal microbiome: Role of proton pump inhibitors. *Current Gastroenterology Reports, 19*(8), 42. https://doi.org/10.1007/s11894-017-0577-6

Mitra, A., MacIntyre, D. A., Lee, Y. S., Smith, A., Marchesi, J. R., Lehne, B., et al. (2015). Cervical intraepithelial neoplasia disease progression is associated with increased vaginal microbiome diversity. *Scientific Reports, 5*, 16865. https://doi.org/10.1038/srep16865

Mitra, A., MacIntyre, D. A., Marchesi, J. R., Lee, Y. S., Bennett, P. R., & Kyrgiou, M. (2016). The vaginal microbiota, human papillomavirus infection and cervical intraepithelial neoplasia: What do we know and where are we going next? *Microbiome, 4*(1), 58. https://doi.org/10.1186/s40168-016-0203-0

Monroy, P. F., Brown, E. H., Sanderson, R. P., Jarrin, G., Mbegbu, M., Kyman, S., & Harris, B. R. (2022). Helicobacter pylori in Native Americans in Northern Arizona. *Diseases, 10*(2), 19. https://doi.org/10.3390/diseases10020019

Monroy, F. P., Brown, H. E., Acevedo-Solis, C. M., Rodriguez-Galaviz, A., Dholakia, R., Pauli, L., & Harris, R. B. (2023). Antibiotic resistance rates for Helicobacter pylori in rural Arizona: A molecular-based study. *Microorganisms, 11*(9). https://doi.org/10.3390/microorganisms11092290

Morales, C. G., Jimenez, N. R., Herbst-Kralovetz, M. M., & Lee, N. R. (2022). Novel vaccine strategies and factors to consider in addressing health disparities of HPV infection and cervical cancer development among Native American women. *Medical Sciences (Basel), 10*(3). https://doi.org/10.3390/medsci10030052

Morton, J. D., Proudfit, J., Calac, D., Portillo, M., Lofton-Fitzsimmons, G., Molina, T., et al. (2013). Creating research capacity through a tribally based institutional review board. *American Journal of Public Health, 103*(12), 2160–2164. https://doi.org/10.2105/AJPH.2013.301473

Munoz, N., Bosch, F. X., de Sanjose, S., Herrero, R., Castellsague, X., Shah, K. V., et al. (2003). Epidemiologic classification of human papillomavirus types associated with cervical cancer. *The New England Journal of Medicine, 348*(6), 518–527. https://doi.org/10.1056/NEJMoa021641

Muslin, C. (2024). Addressing the burden of cervical cancer for Indigenous women in Latin America and the Caribbean: A call for action. *Frontiers in Public Health, 12*, 1376748. https://doi.org/10.3389/fpubh.2024.1376748

Muzny, C. A., Laniewski, P., Schwebke, J. R., & Herbst-Kralovetz, M. M. (2020). Host-vaginal microbiota interactions in the pathogenesis of bacterial vaginosis. *Current Opinion in Infectious Diseases, 33*(1), 59–65. https://doi.org/10.1097/QCO.0000000000000620

NEC. *Cancer among the Navajo 2014–2018*. https://nec.navajo-nsn.gov/Portals/0/Reports/NavajoCancerReport%2013Nov2023.pdf

Norenhag, J., Du, J., Olovsson, M., Verstraelen, H., Engstrand, L., & Brusselaers, N. (2020). The vaginal microbiota, human papillomavirus and cervical dysplasia: A systematic review and network meta-analysis. *BJOG, 127*(2), 171–180. https://doi.org/10.1111/1471-0528.15854

Nugus, P., Desalliers, J., Morales, J., Graves, L., Evans, A., & Macaulay, A. C. (2018). Localizing global medicine: Challenges and opportunities in cervical screening in an indigenous community in Ecuador. *Qualitative Health Research, 28*(5), 800–812. https://doi.org/10.1177/1049732317742129

Oh, H. Y., Kim, B. S., Seo, S. S., Kong, J. S., Lee, J. K., Park, S. Y., et al. (2015). The association of uterine cervical microbiota with an increased risk for cervical intraepithelial neoplasia in Korea. *Clinical Microbiology and Infection, 21*(7), 674 e671–679. https://doi.org/10.1016/j.cmi.2015.02.026

Onywera, H., Williamson, A. L., Mbulawa, Z. Z. A., Coetzee, D., & Meiring, T. L. (2019). The cervical microbiota in reproductive-age South African women with and without human papillomavirus infection. *Papillomavirus Research, 7*, 154–163. https://doi.org/10.1016/j.pvr.2019.04.006

Palleja, A., Mikkelsen, K. H., Forslund, S. K., Kashani, A., Allin, K. H., Nielsen, T., et al. (2018). Recovery of gut microbiota of healthy adults following antibiotic exposure. *Nature Microbiology, 3*(11), 1255–1265. https://doi.org/10.1038/s41564-018-0257-9

Pandey, M. R., & Ernstoff, M. S. (2019). Mechanism of resistance to immune checkpoint inhibitors. *Cancer Drug Resistance, 2*(2), 178–188. https://doi.org/10.20517/cdr.2018.015

Paroni Sterbini, F., Palladini, A., Masucci, L., Cannistraci, C. V., Pastorino, R., Ianiro, G., et al. (2016). Effects of proton pump inhibitors on the gastric mucosa-associated microbiota in dyspeptic patients. *Applied and Environmental Microbiology, 82*(22), 6633–6644. https://doi.org/10.1128/AEM.01437-16

Pete, D., Salama, N. R., Lampe, J. W., Wu, M. C., & Phipps, A. I. (2024). The prevalence and risk factors of Helicobacter pylori infection and cagA virulence gene carriage in adults in the Navajo Nation. *Microbiota in Health and Disease, 6*. https://doi.org/10.26355/mhd_20247_1007

Petrova, M. I., Reid, G., Vaneechoutte, M., & Lebeer, S. (2017). Lactobacillus iners: Friend or foe? *Trends in Microbiology, 25*(3), 182–191. https://doi.org/10.1016/j.tim.2016.11.007

Piyathilake, C. J., Ollberding, N. J., Kumar, R., Macaluso, M., Alvarez, R. D., & Morrow, C. D. (2016). Cervical microbiota associated with higher grade cervical intraepithelial neoplasia in women infected with high-risk human papillomaviruses. *Cancer Prevention Research (Philadelphia, Pa.), 9*(5), 357–366. https://doi.org/10.1158/1940-6207.CAPR-15-0350

Ramirez, J., Guarner, F., Bustos Fernandez, L., Maruy, A., Sdepanian, V. L., & Cohen, H. (2020). Antibiotics as major disruptors of gut microbiota. *Frontiers in Cellular and Infection Microbiology, 10*, 572912. https://doi.org/10.3389/fcimb.2020.572912

Raskov, H., Burcharth, J., & Pommergaard, H. C. (2017). Linking gut microbiota to colorectal cancer. *Journal of Cancer, 8*(17), 3378–3395. https://doi.org/10.7150/jca.20497

Ravel, J., Gajer, P., Abdo, Z., Schneider, G. M., Koenig, S. S., McCulle, S. L., et al. (2011). Vaginal microbiome of reproductive-age women. *Proceedings of the National Academy of Sciences of the United States of America, 108 Suppl 1*(Suppl 1), 4680–4687. https://doi.org/10.1073/pnas.1002611107

Rawla, P., & Barsouk, A. (2019). Epidemiology of gastric cancer: Global trends, risk factors and prevention. *Przegląd Gastroenterologiczny, 14*(1), 26–38. https://doi.org/10.5114/pg.2018.80001

Rawson, A. J. (2024). Anti-racism, racism, and the microbiome: A review. *Progress in Environmental Geography, 3*(2), 137–159. https://doi.org/10.1177/27539687241245428

Rotte, A. (2019). Combination of CTLA-4 and PD-1 blockers for treatment of cancer. *Journal of Experimental & Clinical Cancer Research, 38*(1), 255. https://doi.org/10.1186/s13046-019-1259-z

Sanduleanu, S., Jonkers, D., De Bruine, A., Hameeteman, W., & Stockbrugger, R. W. (2001). Non-Helicobacter pylori bacterial flora during acid-suppressive therapy: Differential findings in gastric juice and gastric mucosa. *Alimentary Pharmacology & Therapeutics, 15*(3), 379–388. https://doi.org/10.1046/j.1365-2036.2001.00888.x

Sankaranarayanan, K., Ozga, T. A., Warinner, C., Tito, Y. R., Obregon-Tito, J. A., Xu, J., et al. (2015). Gut microbiome diversity among Cheyenne and Arapaho individuals from Western Oklahoma. *Current Biology, 25*(24), 3161–3169. https://doi.org/10.1016/j.cub.2015.10.060

Sepich-Poore, D. G., Zitvogel, L., Straussman, R., Hasty, J., Wargo, A. J., & Knight, R. (2021). The microbiome and human cancer. *Science, 371*(6536), eabc4552. https://doi.org/10.1126/science.abc4552

Shah, S. C., Iyer, P. G., & Moss, S. F. (2021). AGA clinical practice update on the management of refractory Helicobacter pylori infection: Expert review. *Gastroenterology, 160*(5), 1831–1841. https://doi.org/10.1053/j.gastro.2020.11.059

Shannon, B., Yi, T. J., Perusini, S., Gajer, P., Ma, B., Humphrys, M. S., et al. (2017). Association of HPV infection and clearance with cervicovaginal immunology and the vaginal microbiota. *Mucosal Immunology, 10*(5), 1310–1319. https://doi.org/10.1038/mi.2016.129

Shulzhenko, N., Lyng, H., Sanson, G. F., & Morgun, A. (2014). Ménage à trois: An evolutionary interplay between human papillomavirus, a tumor, and a woman. *Trends in Microbiology, 22*(6), 345–353. https://doi.org/10.1016/j.tim.2014.02.009

Singh, S., Sharma, P., Sarma, D., Kumawat, M., Tiwari, R., Verma, V., et al. (2023). Implication of obesity and gut microbiome dysbiosis in the etiology of colorectal cancer. *Cancers, 15*(6), 1913. https://doi.org/10.3390/cancers15061913

Sokale, I. O., Thrift, A. P., Montealegre, J., Adekanmbi, V., Chido-Amajuoyi, O. G., Amuta, A., et al. (2023). Geographic variation in late-stage cervical cancer diagnosis. *JAMA Network Open, 6*(11), e2343152. https://doi.org/10.1001/jamanetworkopen.2023.43152

Stebbins, R. C., Noppert, G. A., Aiello, A. E., Cordoba, E., Ward, J. B., & Feinstein, L. (2019). Persistent socioeconomic and racial and ethnic disparities in pathogen burden in the United States, 1999–2014. *Epidemiology and Infection, 147*, e301. https://doi.org/10.1017/S0950268819001894

Story, M., Evans, M., Fabsitz, R. R., Clay, E. T., Rock, H. B., & Broussard, B. (1999). The epidemic of obesity in American Indian communities and the need for childhood obesity-prevention programs. *The American Journal of Clinical Nutrition, 69*(4), 747S–754S. https://doi.org/10.1093/ajcn/69.4.747S

Trinidad, B. S., Blacksher, E., Woodbury, B. R., Hopkins, E. S., Burke, W., Woodahl, L. E., et al. (2022). Precision medicine research with American Indian and Alaska Native communities: Results of a deliberative engagement with tribal leaders. *Genetics in Medicine, 24*(3), 622–630. https://doi.org/10.1016/j.gim.2021.11.003

Usyk, M., Zolnik, C. P., Castle, P. E., Porras, C., Herrero, R., Gradissimo, A., et al. (2020). Cervicovaginal microbiome and natural history of HPV in a longitudinal study. *PLoS Pathogens, 16*(3), e1008376. https://doi.org/10.1371/journal.ppat.1008376

Vinay, D. S., Ryan, E. P., Pawelec, G., Talib, W. H., Stagg, J., Elkord, E., et al. (2015). Immune evasion in cancer: Mechanistic basis and therapeutic strategies. *Seminars in Cancer Biology, 35 Suppl*, S185–S198. https://doi.org/10.1016/j.semcancer.2015.03.004

Vohlonen, I., Pukkala, E., Malila, N., Harkonen, M., Hakama, M., Koistinen, V., & Sipponen, P. (2016). Risk of gastric cancer in Helicobacter pylori infection in a 15-year follow-up. *Scandinavian Journal of Gastroenterology, 51*(10), 1159–1164. https://doi.org/10.1080/00365521.2016.1183225

von Rosenvinge, E. C., Song, Y., White, J. R., Maddox, C., Blanchard, T., & Fricke, W. F. (2013). Immune status, antibiotic medication and pH are associated with changes in the stomach fluid microbiota. *The ISME Journal, 7*(7), 1354–1366. https://doi.org/10.1038/ismej.2013.33

Wang, H., Ma, Y., Li, R., Chen, X., Wan, L., & Zhao, W. (2019). Associations of cervicovaginal lactobacilli with high-risk human papillomavirus infection, cervical intraepithelial neoplasia, and cancer: A systematic review and meta-analysis. *The Journal of Infectious Diseases, 220*(8), 1243–1254. https://doi.org/10.1093/infdis/jiz325

Warbrick, I., Heke, D., & Breed, M. (2023). Indigenous knowledge and the microbiome-bridging the disconnect between colonized places, peoples, and the unseen influences that shape our health and well-being. *mSystems, 8*(1), e0087522. https://doi.org/10.1128/msystems.00875-22

Weinstock, H., Berman, S., & Cates, W., Jr. (2004). Sexually transmitted diseases among American youth: Incidence and prevalence estimates, 2000. *Perspectives on Sexual and Reproductive Health, 36*(1), 6–10. https://doi.org/10.1363/psrh.36.6.04

Weir, H. K., Jim, M. A., Marrett, L. D., & Fairley, T. (2008). Cancer in American Indian and Alaska Native young adults (ages 20–44 years): US, 1999–2004. *Cancer, 113*(5 Suppl), 1153–1167. https://doi.org/10.1002/cncr.23731

White, M. C., Espey, D. K., Swan, J., Wiggins, C. L., Eheman, C., & Kaur, J. S. (2014). Disparities in cancer mortality and incidence among American Indians and Alaska Natives in the United States. *American Journal of Public Health, 104 Suppl 3*(Suppl 3), S377–S387. https://doi.org/10.2105/AJPH.2013.301673

Whop, L. J., Smith, M. A., Butler, T. L., Adcock, A., Bartholomew, K., Goodman, M. T., et al. (2021). Achieving cervical cancer elimination among indigenous women. *Preventive Medicine, 144*, 106314. https://doi.org/10.1016/j.ypmed.2020.106314

Winer, R. L., Gonzales, A. A., Noonan, C. J., Cherne, S. L., Buchwald, D. S., & Collaborative to Improve Native Cancer Outcomes (CINCO). (2016). Assessing acceptability of self-sampling kits, prevalence, and risk factors for human papillomavirus infection in American Indian women. *Journal of Community Health, 41*(5), 1049–1061. https://doi.org/10.1007/s10900-016-0189-3

Xie, N., Shen, G., Gao, W., Huang, Z., Huang, C., & Fu, L. (2023). Neoantigens: Promising targets for cancer therapy. *Signal Transduction and Targeted Therapy, 8*(1), 9. https://doi.org/10.1038/s41392-022-01270-x

Xu, L., Surathu, A., Raplee, I., Chockalingam, A., Stewart, S., Walker, L., et al. (2020). The effect of antibiotics on the gut microbiome: A metagenomics analysis of microbial shift and gut antibiotic resistance in antibiotic treated mice. *Bmc Genomics, 21*(1), 263. https://doi.org/10.1186/s12864-020-6665-2

Yin, Q., Wu, L., Han, L., Zheng, X., Tong, R., Li, L., et al. (2023). Immune-related adverse events of immune checkpoint inhibitors: A review. *Frontiers in Immunology, 14*, 1167975. https://doi.org/10.3389/fimmu.2023.1167975

Yu, L., Lanqing, G., Huang, Z., Xin, X., Minglin, L., Fa-Hui, L., et al. (2023). T cell immunotherapy for cervical cancer: Challenges and opportunities. *Frontiers in Immunology, 14*, 1105265. https://doi.org/10.3389/fimmu.2023.1105265

Yunle, K., Tong, W., Jiyang, L., & Guojun, W. (2024). Advances in Helicobacter pylori vaccine research: From candidate antigens to adjuvants—A review. *Helicobacter, 29*(1). https://doi.org/10.1111/hel.13034

Zamani, M., Ebrahimtabar, F., Zamani, V., Miller, W. H., Alizadeh-Navaei, R., Shokri-Shirvani, J., & Derakhshan, M. H. (2018). Systematic review with meta-analysis: The worldwide prevalence of Helicobacter pylori infection. *Alimentary Pharmacology & Therapeutics, 47*(7), 868–876. https://doi.org/10.1111/apt.14561

Zheng, D., Liwinski, T., & Elinav, E. (2020). Interaction between microbiota and immunity in health and disease. *Cell Research, 30*(6), 492–506. https://doi.org/10.1038/s41422-020-0332-7

Zhou, Z. W., Long, H. Z., Cheng, Y., Luo, H. Y., Wen, D. D., & Gao, L. C. (2021). From microbiome to inflammation: The key drivers of cervical cancer. *Frontiers in Microbiology, 12*, 767931. https://doi.org/10.3389/fmicb.2021.767931

Cancer Health and Indigenous Sexual and Gender Minorities

Josie Raphaelito, Lenny Hayes, and Dornell Pete

Abstract In this chapter, you will learn about the current and developing cancer health landscape as it intersects with Indigenous sexual and gender minority (SGM) populations, including Two-Spirit and Indigenous lesbian, gay, bisexual, transgender, queer, and another identity (LGBTQ+) communities. Background information and Indigenous Knowledge sharing is provided to build understanding of Indigenous gender spectrums, cancer health disparities among Indigenous populations, LGBTQ+ cancer health disparities, and Indigenous SGM health and cancer health disparities. The chapter is authored by Indigenous community leaders and researchers who identify in the Two-Spirit and Native LGBTQ+ communities and provides perspectives on challenges faced by SGM populations, emerging efforts to address SGM cancer health as well as recommendations for building equity and fairness for Indigenous SGM populations for future generations.

Keywords Two-Spirit · Sexual and gender minority cancer health · Indigenous · American Indian · Alaska Native · Native American · Native LGBTQ+ · Sexual and gender minority populations · Lesbian · Gay · Bisexual · Transgender · Queer · Intersex · Asexual · Sexual and gender minority health

---

J. Raphaelito (✉)
Department of Indigenous Cancer Health, Roswell Park Comprehensive Cancer Center, Buffalo, NY, USA
e-mail: Josie.Raphaelito@RoswellPark.org

L. Hayes
Tate Topa Consulting, LLC, Mounds View, MN, USA

D. Pete
Epidemiology Program, Public Health Sciences Division, Fred Hutchinson Cancer Center, Seattle, WA, USA

R. C. Haring (ed.), *Indigenous Genetics, Biobanking, Chemistry, and Cancer Research*, Cancer Health Disparities, https://doi.org/10.1007/978-3-032-17296-9_4

1 Foreword

Before colonization, Two-Spirit and Native LGBTQ+ individuals were honored, respected, and regarded as sacred beings due to the important roles they played within Native American communities. These roles included being name-givers, matchmakers, dreamers, and individuals who could foresee the future and others. However, history shows that the effects of colonization, historical and intergenerational trauma have led to the ostracization of these once-respected individuals within tribal communities. Today, they often represent a forgotten and underserved population.

Evidence indicates a significant lack of data regarding health disparities that affect the Two-Spirit and Native LGBTQ+ community. Often, when data are collected, findings are presented from the perspective of those who do not identify as Two-Spirit or Native LGBTQ+. This disconnect can deter individuals from coming forward to share their health experiences or issues. Therefore, it is crucial to include individuals who identify as Two-Spirit or Native LGBTQ+ in collecting, analyzing, and communicating the results of any health data—including data related to cancer health. It is also important to create safer spaces when asking Two-Spirit and Native LGBTQ+ to participate in any data collection. We must work as community members to be role models for our youth and future generations. Non-Native individuals will not truly understand the impact of historical and intergenerational trauma on the community, but they must work toward a better understanding. Ultimately, Two-Spirit and Native LGBTQ+ leaders and communities work individually and collectively to restore balance, beauty, and acceptance within our tribal communities.

2 Introduction

Two-Spirit is a contemporary umbrella term that was created and defined in the 1990s during Gay American Indian (GAI) organizing among American Indians and Alaska Natives (AI/AN). These Indigenous individuals identified in the mainstream Lesbian, Gay, Bisexual, Transgender, Queer/Questioning community (LGBTQ+), but also understood the notion of more traditional or precontact notions of gender and community roles. This term was created by Indigenous peoples for Indigenous peoples. More specifically, those who identify as Two-Spirit have an understanding and connection to their Indigenous identity, spirituality, and language as it relates to their Native Nation's teachings on diverse gender and sexuality identity spectrums (Fixico, 2020). It should also be noted that not all Indigenous people who identify as LGBTQ+ would also identify as Two-Spirit, and similarly, not all Two-Spirit identifying people would identify as LGBTQ+. It is important to respect an individual's perspective and teachings on Indigenous genders and intersectionality of identities. *Terminology:* Native American, American Indian (AI), and Indigenous are used interchangeably in this chapter. The chapter will also use Two-Spirit and Native LGBTQ+ to acknowledge both Two-Spirit and Native Americans who identify within LGBTQ+ communities.

What is equally important to know is that Two-Spirit and Indigenous LGBTQ+ individuals have always been part of Indigenous communities and have even been documented in settler contact records. Indigenous communities are healing from external and lateral violence that specifically targets Two-Spirit (2S) and Native LGBTQ+ community members. Healing often begins with learning about Two-Spirit ancestors, acknowledging Indigenous Knowledge as it relates to genders, and building an understanding of today's Two-Spirit and Native LGBTQ+ relatives. We know there is strength in culture and language reclamation across Indian Country, including recovering and/or rebuilding teachings and understandings of traditional gender roles, gender spectrums, and acknowledging that individuals who identify in today's lesbian, gay, bisexual, transgender, queer, intersex communities were present and resilient in precolonial existence.

These traditional gender and sexual orientation spectrums vary across Native Nations. When aiming for health equity across Indigenous communities (from children to elders), we should also consider and actively engage relatives who identify on these spectrums, so we can build a more fair and accessible healthcare system for everyone. Historically, Two-Spirit and LGBTQI+ (I, intersex) populations have reported higher discrimination than non-LGBTQI individuals (Parker, 2017). Two-Spirit and Native LGBTQ+ relatives continue to face systemic challenges, including policies specifically targeting trans and gender nonconforming individuals that pose risks to health and well-being, intensifying the challenges our Two-Spirit and Native LGBTQ+ relatives endure—ranging from violence and trauma to rejection and denial of critical healthcare services. In this chapter, you will learn about the current and developing cancer health landscape as it intersects with Two-Spirit and Indigenous LGBTQ+ communities.

On the Navajo Nation and in Albuquerque, NM, Diné/Native LGBTQ2S+ relatives gathered around meals, sharing laughter, stories, and reflections as they had for generations. In these moments of connection, we discussed our identities and the often painful challenges—family rejection, discrimination in healthcare, and unrelenting struggles for acceptance. Words once considered taboo—'Transgender,' 'Queer,' 'Same-sex marriage,' and 'Nadleeh'—now flowed freely as part of our shared dialogue in our Native LGBTQA2S+ support group.

As the stories brought laughter and tears, they brought to light a general avoidance of healthcare use and timely treatment due to a lack of safe, culturally appropriate, and affirming healthcare. One transwoman joked that one way to get healthcare was to just go to jail or prison. Transgender people overall have higher rates of incarceration and transgender people of color have even higher rates. However, the correctional system is highly gender segregated and a quarter of transgender inmates are denied access to healthcare. This experience can be found among many of our Native LGBTQA2S+ relatives.—Personal story and observation from Dr. Dornell Pete, Diné

3 Cancer Health Disparities Among AI/AN People

Through a public health framework, this chapter considers drivers of cancer disparities as key indicators for cancer health outcomes among AI/AN who identify in the Two-Spirit and LGBTQIA+ communities. In an effort to communicate the people and specific areas in need of support, the US public health system measures factors related to *Social Drivers of Health (SDOH)*, for which data are collected on the following topics: education level; income; employment; housing; transportation; and access to healthy food, clean air, water, and healthcare services. Additional considerations for drivers of health include lived experience (including lack of trust with medical institutions) and various other biological and environmental factors (American Association for Cancer Research, 2024). The 2024 Cancer Disparities report from the American Association for Cancer Research provides a great overview and description of contributing factors for cancer disparities, which include racism, discrimination, structural inequities, and social injustices; all of which could have a double impact on Indigenous people who also identify as Two-Spirit and/or within the LGBTQ+ communities.

When evaluating SDOH indicators across communities and Tribal Nations, apparent disparities can be identified when comparing AI/AN populations to non-Hispanic, White people (NHW). When we look at life expectancy between both populations, we see that the life expectancy of AI/AN people is lower than NWH people (65.6 years vs. 76.7 years) (Arias et al., 2023). The highest mortality rates include unintentional injuries, heart disease, and cancer for AI/AN people across the United States (Arias et al., 2023).

As cancer is the second leading cause of death for AI/AN people in the United States, a better understanding of cancer in Indigenous communities is imperative. A 2024 article, the Landmark Series: Surgical Oncology Care in Native Americans—The Indian Health Service (Huyser, 2025), provides an overview of cancer incidence and cancer-related mortality among AI/ANs while also providing historical context to the Indian Health Service as an important healthcare delivery system for AI/ANs here in the United States. Major cancer health disparities highlighted in this article include:

- AI/ANs have the highest overall cancer incidence and highest cancer mortality compared with all races.
- When diagnosed with cancer at the same stage as NHW patients, AI/ANs patients have a 10% lower 5-year survival rate.
- Lung, liver, stomach, kidney, uterine, and colorectal cancer incidence rates are twice as high among AI/ANs compared with NHWs.
- Risk of cancer death is 51% higher for AI/ANs than NHWs when adjusting for stage, sex, and age.

Major risk factors contributing to high cancer incidence and mortality rates among AI/ANs include lack of access to cancer care and screening, limited transportation to access prevention and intervention services, increased environmental exposures to carcinogens, and lack of trust in health systems due to historical and intergenerational traumas, among others.

4 Intersectionality and Health Disparities

Why would we look at cancer disparities as it relates to race, gender, and sexuality? Because a person's sexual orientation and gender identity can influence or compound an individual's cancer risk factors. Understanding the intersections of Indigenous, sexual orientation, and gender helps public health professionals, healthcare providers, and researchers to tailor health promotion and prevention efforts that speak to the Two-Spirit and Indigenous LGBTQ+ population, provide patient-centered quality healthcare, and create research space that builds cancer health knowledge as it relates to an often-invisible population.

Intersectionality is a theoretical framework developed by Kimberle Crenshaw to understand how multiple social identities, such as race, gender, sexual orientation, and disability, intersect at the individual level, reflecting systems of privilege and oppression (Cho, 2013). Through this framework, race, gender, and sexual orientation interact to share the multiple dimensions of Two-Spirit and Indigenous LGBTQ+ health experiences. Intersectionality makes it clear that people of intersectional identities experience outcomes like cancer that are distinct from a single identity. And if we ignore this intersection, we lose understanding of important differences in the experiences of adverse health outcomes.

Homophobia, racism, and heterosexism are the resulting systems of the intersection we speak about for Two-Spirit and Indigenous LGBTQ+, creating complex layers of oppression that must be understood together. Public health professionals, providers, and researchers must use an intersectionality framework to understand health inequities and challenge single and binary paradigms, i.e., "those working through an intersectional lens illustrate how identity is linked to multiple vectors of power." (Balestrery, 2012). This approach is holistic in identifying root causes to ill-health, including cancer, as well as achieving wellness for the Two-Spirit and Native LGBTQ+ population. We must also make efforts in our work to understand how colonialism is linked to cancer risk, as Indigenous people are living in a legacy of centuries of colonialism.

The rich history of Two-Spirit and Native LGBTQ+ people, woven through generations of storytelling, is a testament to our strength, survival, and cultural significance. Despite centuries of erasure, our identities continue to thrive, supported by the resilience of our ancestors and elders. According to the Williams Institute, there are an estimated 285,000 AI/AN adults in the United States who identify as LGBTQ, which is about 6% of the total AI/AN population. We know these numbers will grow over generations as people accept and feel comfortable with their identities. Many still speak their language and practice their cultural ways and traditions. They depend on generations of teachings and stories for survival and living in harmony with the land and one another.

5 Sexual and Gender Minority Health

There is developing research and data available to more accurately describe health disparities among sexual and gender minority (SGM) populations when compared to heterosexual and cisgender populations, but more work to collect data on the health of SGM people is needed. The most recent Gallup Poll for population estimates showed that individuals who identify with LGBTQ+ communities increased in the United States, and the value now stands at 7.6% (up from 5.6% in 2020). The Gallup Poll (n = 12,000 Americans aged 18+) also found that more than one in five adults who are from Generation Z (born in the late 1990s) identify as LGBTQ+ (Jones, 2024). Gallup's first poll measuring sexual orientation and transgender identity was in 2012. These data trends suggest that younger generations are twice as likely as the previous generations to identify as LGBTQ+. This growing population will require more out of a public health system, such as cultural competency training for clinical and patient facing staff; adapted and targeted education materials; group focused outreach and engagement initiatives; clarifications for cancer screening eligibility criteria with inclusive language; representation at policy and decision-making levels; and inclusive career pathways to public health and STEAM (science, technology, engineering, arts, and mathematics) fields.

> *Lifetime exposure to interpersonal stressors like stigma, discrimination, and violence as well as structural stressors like anti-LGBTQ+ public policies engender poor health outcomes among LGBTQ+ adults.* (Fredriksen-Goldsen et al., 2014; Fredriksen-Goldsen & de Vries, 2019; Lampe et al., 2024)

Resources such as the Behavioral Risk Factor Surveillance System (BRFSS) collect state data about the health behaviors and status of US adults, including adults who identify as LGBTQ+. Highlights include the following:

- BRFSS data from 2014 to 2017 found that LGBTQ+ adults have higher rates of poverty compared with their counterparts. Bisexual cisgender women and transgender people had the highest poverty rates.
- BRFSS data from 2015 to 2018 found that older LGBTQ+ adults (45 years and older) were more likely to report subjective cognitive decline (i.e., Alzheimer's disease and related dementias), which has been connected to chronic minority stress experienced over a lifetime.
- Other chronic health conditions such as cardiovascular disease and some cancers can be correlated to high levels of substance and alcohol misuse among SGM populations.

A 2021 national LGBTQ+ survey with Black, Indigenous, and People of Color (BIPOC) respondents found similar to BRFSS results. Cancer-related behaviors such as alcohol consumption (52% BIPOC vs. 45% White) and poor mental health (92% BIPOC vs. 83% White) were found to be higher among BIPOC survey respondents than those in White respondents. Respondents stated that LGBTQ+ tailored resources (health education brochures, visibility, acknowledgment in media campaigns, etc.) are very important to address risky health behaviors.

To capture the perspectives of healthcare providers, an annual report created by the National Coalition for LGBTQ Health engaged more than 1000 providers to explore the state of LGBTQ+ health through a national survey (National Coalition for LGBTQ Health, 2023). Major findings from the report are outlined as follows:

- Providers understand the barriers LGBTQ individuals face in accessing healthcare to be linked to pervasive stigma, a lack of trust in the healthcare system, healthcare costs, and challenges to accessing health insurance.
- There is a need for more training to help providers understand the stigma experienced by LGBTQ patients and create more inclusive spaces.
- Providers identified advocacy priorities centered on LGBTQ equality, stronger gender-affirming care protections, and identifying affordable housing for LGBTQ patients.
- Providers also recognized the importance of recruiting compassionate staff, providing comprehensive and inclusive training, and coordinating and learning from providers experienced in working with LBGTQ patients.

SGM Cancer Health Data Many organizations, institutes, and local and regional entities now collect and organize SGM cancer health data. Advocates and SGM health leaders have hosted multitudes of trainings and technical assistance to build understanding and provide tools for cancer hospitals and care coordinators to better serve SGM patients and families. Although January 2025 Executive Orders have begun to strip away SGM patient's rights to accessing care and have removed SGM data from portals such as the National Institutes of Health and the Centers for Disease Control and Prevention, organizations such as the National LGBT Cancer Network continue to organize and fight for strategies to archive SGM cancer datasets, reports, manuscripts, and other SGM cancer research work from the past few decades. With support from the SGM cancer researcher field, this important work will prevail and SGM populations will not be erased.

The National LGBT Cancer Network is also responsible for the 2021 national report titled, "Out: The National Cancer Survey." Data were collected from 1200 cancer survivors to deepen understanding among healthcare leaders of LGBT experiences with cancer. A supplemental report specific to the LGBTQ+ BIPOC cancer journey builds further knowledge needed within cancer care networks. Key findings from that BIPOC survey include:

- The top five cancers among respondents were breast cancer, prostate, colorectal, anal, and skin cancer.
- The median age at diagnosis was 49, and 30% of respondents were diagnosed at 51–60.
- Respondents were more likely to experience negative encounters during cancer diagnosis, care, and treatment. Accessing culturally competent providers was reported as more difficult.
- Respondents were two times as likely to be dissatisfied with cancer treatment experiences compared with White and Latinx respondents.

- Health settings were described as less welcoming after disclosing LGBTQ+ identity compared with White respondents.

6 Two-Spirit and Native LGBTQ Populations and Cancer Health

Research consistently shows that LGBTQ individuals, particularly those who are uninsured or marginalized, face significant barriers to cancer screenings and care. For Two-Spirit and Native LGBTQ+ relatives, these disparities are even more pronounced, with historical trauma, mistrust of healthcare systems, and lack of culturally relevant care creating compounding obstacles. In addition, the absence of sexual orientation and gender identity (SOGI) data for Two-Spirit and Native LGBTQ+ people masks the inequities and prevents us from understanding their unmet needs; additionally, this hinders the development, monitoring, and evaluation of healthcare systems and targeted interventions.

Unfortunately, data on the health and healthcare experiences of Two-Spirit and Native LGBTQ+ populations are extremely limited, particularly when it comes to cancer prevention, screening, and care. The limited research available indicates that Two-Spirit and Native LGBTQ+ community members encounter more challenges when seeking cancer care (Kamen et al., 2019; Boehmer et al., 2014). There is a lack of representation of Two-Spirit and Native LGBTQ+ people in cancer education research among the SGM population, which needs to be addressed with outreach and inclusion efforts. Inclusion of Two-Spirit and Native LGBTQ+ people is not only vitally important in the community outreach setting, but it is also considered an emerging area of importance within the SGM cancer health realm.

Upon further analysis of cancer health data and Indigenous SGM landscapes, we see that there is a lack of Indigenous SGM awareness among cancer health providers and community health outreach specialists. A study conducted in 2023 via online surveys identified barriers to care among LGBTQ+ and Two-Spirit American Indians and Alaska Natives (Hoover, 2023). This study showed that gender-diverse individuals in particular encountered barriers to care at a greater proportion than their cisgender counterparts, such as higher reports of providers refusing care (48.2% vs. 31.0%: $P = 0.006$), providers being inadequately trained in Two-Spirit care, fear of negative community perceptions of gender diverse individuals, and greater financial insecurity. In addition, all groups of Two-Spirit and LGBTQ+ individuals faced difficulties in accessing care due to traveling long distances and faced higher barriers to access to care compared with the general AI/AN population.

Moreover, research with the LGBTQ+ population more broadly indicates that there is reason to believe that Two-Spirit and Native LGBTQ+ people are at greater risk for developing cancer, as well as experiencing suboptimal engagement with cancer education and screening to reduce their risks. Roswell Park Comprehensive Cancer Center's Department of Indigenous Cancer Health led a quality improvement project engaging Two-Spirit and Native LGBTQ+ community members in virtual roundtable discussions to receive feedback and guidance on adaptations needed to cancer health education materials. Themes around the importance of representation in outreach materials; gender diverse language, communal health, and sincere acknowledgment of heritage and identity emerged from these discussions. This feedback continues to be utilized during education material development within the department and shared with partners to promote inclusion and respect for SGM relatives.

With careful maneuvering around anti-diversity, equity, and inclusion (DEI) federal policies and executive orders, many cancer health outreach and engagement initiatives are continuing to expand their community reach to best meet the needs of their service area. This book and this chapter provide insightful background and rational around the need to not only engage Indigenous partners to strengthen cancer health outreach efforts but also the opportunities to support Indigenous SGM populations. We need to continue listening and learning about barriers to cancer healthcare for Indigenous SGM communities, including intergenerational and historical traumas stemming from structural systems that continue to infiltrate their healthcare needs.

Decolonize the Cancer Research Approach We need to decolonize our approach to collect more meaningful data to understand the disparities and resiliencies in Two-Spirit and Native LGBTQ+ people. The first step is understanding that our current health metrics were established within dominant frameworks. Maggie Walter and Chris Anderson posit, "many of these data, as they currently exist, tend to constitute Indigenous peoples as deficient and that these portrayals can, and do, restrict and inhibit other ways of understanding or using statistical data by, and for, Indigenous peoples." (Walter & Andersen, 2013). Deficit-based approaches misrepresent groups and perpetuate negative stereotypes and racism.

How do we decolonize this approach? We can utilize Indigenous Health Frameworks such as cultural value-based systems, seventh generation philosophy to create long-lasting impact into future generations, and connections to land environment to introduce and define more meaningful, measurable ways to understand cancer risk among our Two-Spirit and Native LGBTQ+ relatives. These frameworks inform how to center our knowledge systems, worldviews, and context to bring change in our health outcomes.

Dr. Dornell Pete's research relied heavily on the Diné concept of Ké (Navajo translation: kinship) to identify data that measures the relationality between the person (including SOGI data), kin, and environment. For example, in Dr. Pete's Navajo Stomach Study, she/they developed questions to ask study participants about modifiable factors related to stomach cancer, such as consuming traditional foods, practicing traditional ways, participating in tribal ceremonies, and living off the land. The study ensured that these data had input from the community and aligned with tribal values related to connectedness to land, cultural continuity, and identity, which represents an important strengths-based approach to quantifying the degree Diné people are connected to their culture and how that we may identify positive aspects of their health to counter stomach cancer risk. These data were not only meaningful to the tribe when Dr. Pete disseminated results back to the community, but it allowed her/them to change the narrative through her/their writing and speaking about stomach cancer risk among Diné people. This example highlights a path to decolonize the data and cancer research approach.

Data on the strengths and resilience of Two-Spirit and Native LGBTQ+ people is scarce. Therefore, this is the time for tribes and Native researchers, programming, and healthcare systems to collect Native health data based on their traditional knowledge systems and histories and the impact on health and well-being.

7 Emerging Efforts in Cancer Health and SGM

This chapter was drafted in the Fall of 2024. Since then, many things have changed in the United States for SGMs and individuals from the expansive LGBTQ+ communities. Most notably, there is a national effort being led by the federal government to roll back decades of advocacy, human rights policy and law, and inclusion efforts to build health equity for SGM populations. This section will provide an update on the current landscape and impact of White House executive orders on SGM health. More importantly, this section will also provide a brief description of foundational work that will continue in the wake of attempts to dismantle and erase a proud and strong LGBTQ+ population in the United States, including Two-Spirit and Native LGBTQ+ communities.

Provided below is a general timeline and summary of major directives made to federal agencies because of US Presidential Executive Orders issued in January 2025.

- January 29, 2025, federal agencies such as the Centers for Disease Control and Prevention (CDC) received notice to implement executive orders entitled *Ending Radical and Wasteful Government DEI Programs and Preferencing and Initial Rescissions of Harmful Executive Orders and Action*—including immediate termination of all programs, personnel, activities, or contracts promoting diversity, equity, and inclusion.
- January 31, 2025, the US Department of Health and Human Services received notice to implement executive orders entitled *Defending Women from Gender Ideology Extremism and Restoring Biological Truth to the Federal Government*—essentially, this was an anti-trans and anti-SGM push from the federal government as it relates to programs, personnel, activities, contracts, and research supported by federal funds.
- January 31, 2025 is the deadline issued by the US Office of Personnel Management to comply with "Defending Women" executive orders by terminating any programs that promote gender ideology; taking down all outward facing media that promotes gender ideology; removing pronouns from email signature lines; cancelling training promoting SGM inclusion; updating all agency forms to list male

or female only and not gender identity or option to enter "sex"; and removal of SGM data from federal agency websites.

Foundational SGM Health Efforts Prior to January 2025, the US health systems were expanding inclusion efforts to better serve the growing SGM populations. Although federal policy and the dismantling of diversity, equity, and inclusion efforts make health equity strategies more difficult, there are many foundational frameworks in place to support SGM populations moving forward. Examples of foundational SGM health efforts through a public health lens that help meet the cancer health needs of LGBTQ+ populations are provided as follows.

- *Policy and advocacy*: Organizing and network building have strengthened over the past few decades and strong advocacy efforts continue to emerge. National, regional, local, and tribal advocates are proving their allyship and joining or even leading policy and advocacy efforts to ensure Two-Spirit and LGBTQ+ communities are not erased. Policy and laws such as New York State's Civil rights laws prohibit discrimination on the basis of sex, sexual orientation, gender identity, gender expression, or disability. Collectively, policy and law makers and advocates will continue to take action and utilize existing frameworks and pathways to protect LGBTQ+ rights.
- *Health protection*: SGM health certifications are available across North America for hospitals and clinics to denote when their teams (from receptionists to healthcare providers) are trained in health equity and inclusion and when their institute is designated as "safe." For example, Roswell Park Comprehensive Cancer Center—an NCI-designated Cancer Center—located on traditional Haudenosaunee land in Buffalo, NY, has been designated as a leader on the Health Equity Index from the Human Rights Campaign to amplify their cancer center's efforts to build understanding and a safer space for SGM communities to access cancer healthcare.
- *Health improvement*: The development and implementation of cultural competency training made available to health systems and organizations is an ongoing strategy to create safer spaces and understanding of SGM health needs. Additionally, cultural competency training specific to Indigenous populations that draws connections to the intersection of identities and identifies opportunities to create more fair and accessible healthcare services for Two-Spirit and Native LGBTQ+ populations is available/needed.
- *Assessment and surveillance*: Leaders in cancer research and cancer disparities such as the American Association of Cancer Research recognize the lack of SOGI data but also encourage national cancer registries and other health records to routinely collect and document SOGI data to develop a more comprehensive snapshot of cancer incidence and mortality among SGM individuals. Yet, there are realistic fears that SOGI data could be used for harm. Protection of SOGI data should consider the concerns of the small Native LGBTQ+ population, and if patients or participants opt in for sharing their SOGI data, their information must be secured through HIPAA/state/tribal data privacy laws that require disclosure of the patient to share information with federal and outside entities.

- *Research*: Research goes hand in hand with SOGI data. The lack of population-level SOGI data prevents researchers from understanding the health disparities in the SGM population and identifying strategies or interventions to target. Research on SGM health across the lifespan has shown high burdens of HIV, sexually transmitted infections (STI), STI-related cancers, and mental health conditions (Lampe, 2023). Yet, more SGM health research is needed on the causes of these disease burdens, such as tobacco, alcohol, and substance use, as well as on barriers to accessing healthcare and public health interventions. Prior to 2024, the National Institutes of Health (NIH) designated the SGM population as a group with health disparities and, therefore, a group to focus on. As a result, NIH established the Sexual and Gender Minority Research Office to support and coordinate SGM research across multiple institutes. However, this new administration terminated this office and federal funding for the SGM population. These major setbacks have led to private foundations filling this funding gap, which can be found within an academic or research institution or from donors or private corporations.

Promising Two-Spirit and Native LGBTQ+ Endeavors The resources provided below may be limited, unavailable, or terminated due to the 2025 Executive Orders from the White House. This chapter applauds their efforts and presents them as promising endeavors for Tribal Nations to support. These resources could be revitalized by Tribal Nations and their cancer health systems as an act of tribal sovereignty and meeting the needs of all their Tribal Nation's citizens.

- *Tribal data sovereignty*: Data can drive change, inform critical decisions, and direct the allocation of resources—yet for many Native communities, data have often been used to reinforce colonial frameworks and perpetuate harm. Fortunately, Tribes are becoming knowledgeable about this. This has empowered Tribes to exert their tribal sovereign right to critique, collect, and own data. Many tribes are taking steps to understand what health metrics are needed to describe the health of their population, determine health priorities, set health policies, and protect their people. Native researchers are also theorizing and employing innovative approaches to characterize Native health through quantitative and qualitative methods founded on empirical, traditional, and revealed knowledge systems (LaFrance & Nichols, 2008).
- *Tribal health programs and tribal organizations*: The Northwest Portland Area Indian Health Board launched a second addition to their toolkit titled "Celebrating Our Magic" in early 2025. This resource is designed to support Two-Spirit, Native transgender, and gender diverse youth, families, and healthcare providers. The toolkit helps identify strategies to increase access to care, create better gender-affirming clinical environments, and support positive mental health outcomes. This type of resource can be shared with other clinical settings, such as cancer care environments and cancer centers, to further support Two-Spirit and Native LBGTQ+ patients and families. Additionally, tribes are developing their own cancer control plans, which aim to reduce cancer rates by setting goals and

identifying strategies for intervention. Addressing Two-Spirit and Native LGBTQ+ equity as a key dimension in these plans is essential.

- *Networking and gathering*: The "Science of Cancer Health Equity in Sexual and Gender Minority Communities" gathering is an annual cancer health research summit hosted by SGM cancer leaders from across the country. This space was created to highlight SGM cancer health work (research, data collection, community engagement, etc.) and promote networking and develop expertise. Research specific to Two-Spirit and Native LGBTQ+ cancer health have been included in these gatherings and will continue to be part of this gathering.
- *Culturally competent education material*: The American Indian Cancer Foundation developed and continues to distribute cancer health-specific materials with and for Two-Spirit and Native LGBTQ+ communities. Cancer education and screening language has been adapted to meet the needs of gender diverse populations and can be used during any cancer health community outreach and engagement efforts.
- *Inclusive SOGI data*: Various data collection methods and language are developing across healthcare settings as these relate to including SOGI data collection upon patient intake and registration processes. For SOGI data collection, CDISC (Clinical Data Interchange Standards Consortium) is a trusted entity with new recommendations provided in Fall of 2024. For example, CDISC provides templates and guidance on demographic and SOGI questionnaire development for patients to be utilized in healthcare settings. The questionnaire, however, leaves out "Two-Spirit" as an option in gender and sexual orientation and offers a "I use a different term" option.

  Data collected through CDISC is used by the healthcare clinical team to better understand the patient, possible barriers to trust, and help support healthcare equity throughout the process. Depending on tribal, state, and private healthcare policies and law, as well as funding mechanisms (federally, state, tribally, privately run clinics and hospitals), SOGI data from healthcare institutes may be provided to the North American Association of Central Cancer Registries (NAACCR) where data can be accessed and analyzed to understand health disparities of Two-Spirit and Native LGBTQ+ people.
- *National LGBTQ+ collaboration*: The National LGBTQ Cancer Network is a national leader and is organized around educating, training, and advocating for LGBT cancer survivors and those at risk. They are collecting and organizing a compendium of LGBT promising practices across the cancer care continuum, including resources to support cross-cutting issues such as data, workforce, systems, information, and diversity. Their team is traveling out to healthcare settings across the country to educate and inform clinicians, researchers, and community leaders about LGBTQ+ cancer health, as well as national priorities and advocacy efforts. Their leadership is actively involved in national and international discussions related to SGM cancer health, data, research, and health equity. They welcome engagement opportunities with Two-Spirit and Native LGBTQIA+ cancer health initiatives.

- *Emerging ECHO use in the healthcare field*: Prior to the 2025 Executive Orders, the Northwest Portland Area Indian Health Board led an initiative called Indian Country ECHO (Extension for Community Healthcare Outcomes), which creates a community of healthcare professionals practicing in Indian Country. Specifically, ECHO offers telehealth training to build networks, collaborate on case consultations, and create mentorship opportunities with clinical experts serving Indigenous populations. They developed a Trans and Gender Confirming ECHO series with providers in the field working with gender diverse adult patients. Ultimately, Indian Country ECHO helps increase access to specialty care, including trans and gender confirming healthcare needs. This type of ECHO series could expand to include support around cancer screening needs among Two-Spirit and Native LGBTQ+ populations. This is a powerful resource that, if revitalized, could continue to have a positive impact in transgender and gender affirming healthcare practices. https://www.nativehealthresources.org/resource/celebrating-our-magic-toolkit-2/

8 Recommendations for Indigenous SGM and Cancer Health

In addition to rescinding executive orders and anti-SGM practices at the federal level, the following recommendations are provided to continue advancing support for SGM populations and creating safer healthcare settings for all patients. Tribal Nations can utilize tribal sovereignty to maintain or develop policies and law to protect Indigenous SGM populations, and LGBTQ+ protective state laws can also be considered to maintain and build support for SGM cancer health.

- Maintain a momentum of inclusion efforts throughout anticipated SGM health policy changes. When health equity and inclusion are challenged by politics, there is an opportunity to revisit values and missions of cancer health initiatives and services. Align your work with shared values with health organizations and entities that commit to maintaining healthcare services to SGM populations.
- Build understanding of Indigenous populations:
  - Educate your team(s) about Native Nations in your region. Acknowledge the Indigenous lands you occupy, and support efforts to engage within Native Nations. Create meaningful engagement to build trust with Native Nations that fosters outreach, opportunities to learn from one another, support for reciprocity, and pathways to STEAM education and careers.
  - Review and share publications such as "Tribal Nations & the United States: An Introduction" from the National Congress of American Indians to understand the distinct relationships between Native Nations and the Federal Government, especially as it relates to healthcare.

- Institutional policy:
  - Require cultural competency training among all staff.
  - Require collection of SOGI data that includes Two-Spirit as an option.
  - Utilize existing data collection tools such as CDISC for inclusive SOGI data intake forms.
- Epidemiology:
  - Create inclusive community profiles to better measure Social Determinants of Health among SGM populations.
- Outreach and engagement:
  - Partner with Indigenous health experts to develop Indigenous SGM outreach efforts.
  - Invite leaders from Indigenous SGM communities to participate in your institute's "Community Advisory Boards" or other advisory groups to support your work and expand your perspectives.
  - Engage, listen, and learn from existing resources to support SGM populations.
  - Train healthcare providers and staff about how to collect and ethically use SOGI data to better inform healthcare needs.
- Health administration:
  - Promote patient-centered care as a valuable framework to help build trust between patients and healthcare providers.
  - Develop compliance and evaluation processes and procedures to ensure high standards of inclusion of SGM people.
- Health promotion:
  - Encourage simulation training of gender-affirming care for healthcare workers (oncology-specific content).

9 Reflections and Conclusion

The dominant models of delivery of healthcare services in tribal communities are inconsistent with many Native cultures and concepts of health. The United States conceptualizes health linearly. Native concepts of health are circular and focus on at least four domains of well-being, including spirit, body, mind, and context. When these domains interact in balance, health and well-being are the results: "when in harmony, people thrive, are resilient beyond expectation, and contributes synergistically to those around them with their energy." (Hodge et al., 2009; Lavallee & Poole, 2010). Health and wellness involve the person and the balance in tribal communities.

Health, culture, and identity are important at the individual and collective levels. Yet there needs to be openness for restoring health, culture, and identity because a one-size-fits-all does not work when tribal cultures, languages, and identities are unique.

Since time immemorial, tribes have relied on ancestral knowledge, sacred land, traditional foods, medicines, and skills not just to survive but to thrive in the face of adversity. It is frightening to think that healthcare as a public good may not be accessible to everyone, as this far-right administration considers cuts to Medicaid and health research. How certain are we that the responsibility of the United States to provide healthcare to Native people will not disappear?

As Two-Spirit and Queer Indigenous authors and cancer researchers, we have identified ways to be more strategic and respectful in approaches to measure and understand Two-Spirit and Native LGBTQ+ health. We have the opportunity to encourage other Native researchers to break down the cycle of homophobia, heteronormativity, sexism, and racism in our research. We must also recognize unjust processes and practices in institutional and government structures through critical inquiry and questioning and take action.

While we do not have a true understanding of the cancer disparities among Two-Spirit and Native LGBTQ+ populations, these individuals are decolonizing their place in tribal societies by being present in the spaces that exclude them, rooted in culture and associated with their traditions that honor multiple genders. We are excited about where we will go next.

Cancer is preventable and will require creative and innovative steps. In the thoughts of Billy-Ray Belcourt (Driftpil Cree Nation, Poet) (Belcourt, 2016), I am intrigued by going beyond the norm. As Belcourt ingeniously asks, "What would happen if we went wild, if we refused domestication and instead chose lawlessness? When our backs are against the wall, we do not have many options from which to choose. Tradition does biopolitical work: it operates at the level of autonomy, not only reifying gender's collapse into biology but also training our bodies into thinking that we have finally found something that feels like something. I'm not buying it, and I think that queer identity is the point of departure decolonization has been waiting for. It's your move."

Two-Spirit and Native LGBTQ+ people deserve health and wellness
Two-Spirit and Native LGBTQ+ people deserve health and wellness
Two-Spirit and Native LGBTQ+ people deserve health and wellness
Two-Spirit and Native LGBTQ+ people deserve health and wellness….

Acknowledgments The lead author acknowledges past and present Two-Spirit and Native LGBTQ+ relatives who continue to fight for recognition, inclusion, and health equity both within Indigenous and outside of Indigenous communities. She also acknowledges that this chapter contributes to the ever-growing efforts of other Two-Spirit and Native LGBTQ+ relatives whose work is aimed at building inclusive and understanding spaces for generations to come. This work was supported by Roswell Park Comprehensive Cancer Center and National Cancer Institute (NCI) grant P30CA016056; Bristol Meyers Squibb Foundation, Roswell Park Department of Indigenous Cancer Health, Indigenous/Rural Patient Navigation, Fred Hutchinson Cancer Center.

References

American Association for Cancer Research. (2024). *AACR cancer disparities progress report 2024*. Retrieved May 5, 2025 from https://cancerprogressreport.aacr.org/wp-content/uploads/sites/2/2024/05/AACR_CDPR__2024.pdf

Arias, E., Xu, J., & Kochanek, K. (2023). United States Life Tables, 2021. *National vital statistics* reports: *From the Centers for Disease Control and Prevention, National Center* for *Health Statistics. National Vital Statistics System, 72*(12), 1–64.

Balestrery, J. E. (2012). Intersecting discourses on race and sexuality: Compounded colonization among LGBTTQ American Indians/Alaska Natives. *Journal of Homosexuality, 59*(5), 633–655. https://doi.org/10.1080/00918369.2012.673901

Belcourt, B.-R. (2016). A poltergeist manifesto. *Feral Feminisms, 6*(6), 22–32. https://feralfeminisms.com/a-poltergeist-manifesto/

Cho, S., Crenshaw, K. W., & McCall, L. (2013). Toward a field of intersectionality studies: Theory, applications, and praxis. *Signs: Journal of Women in Culture and Society, 38*(4), 785–810.

Fredriksen-Goldsen, K. I., Cook-Daniels, L., Kim, H. J., Erosheva, E. A., Emlet, C. A., Hoy-Ellis, C. P., et al. (2014). Physical and mental health of transgender older adults: An at-risk and underserved population. *Gerontologist, 54*(3), 488–500. https://doi.org/10.1093/geront/gnt021

Hodge, D. R., Limb, G. E., & Cross, T. L. (2009). Moving from colonization toward balance and harmony: A Native American perspective on wellness. *Social Work, 54*(3), 211–219. https://doi.org/10.1093/sw/54.3.211

Huyser, M. R. (2025). The landmark series: Surgical oncology care in Native Americans-the Indian Health Service. *Annals of Surgical Oncology, 32*(4), 2379–2392. https://doi.org/10.1245/s10434-024-16655-1

Jones, J. M. (2024). LGBTQ+ Identification in US Now at 7.6%: more than one in five Gen Z adults identify as LGBTQ+. *Gallup*. https://news.gallup.com/poll/611864/lgbtq-identification.aspx

LaFrance, J., & Nichols, R. (2008). Reframing evaluation: Defining an indigenous evaluation framework. *Canadian Journal of Program Evaluation, 23*(2), 13–31. https://doi.org/10.3138/cjpe.23.003

Lampe, N. M., Barbee, H., Tran, N. M., Bastow, S., & McKay, T. (2024). Health disparities among lesbian, gay, bisexual, transgender, and queer older adults: A structural competency approach. *International Journal of Aging & Human Development, 98*(1), 39–55. https://doi.org/10.1177/00914150231171838

Lavallee, L. F., & Poole, J. M. (2010). Beyond recovery: Colonization, health and healing for indigenous people in Canada. *International Journal of Mental Health and Addiction, 8*(2), 271–281. https://doi.org/10.1007/s11469-009-9239-8

National Coalition for LGBTQ Health. (2023). *State of LGBTQ Health™ Second Annual National Survey*. Retrieved May 5, 2025 from https://healthlgbtq.org/stateof/lgbtqhealth/#introduction

Walter, M., & Andersen, C. (2013). *Indigenous statistics: A quantitative research methodology*. Left Coast Press. https://doi.org/10.4324/9781315426570

Surgery Data in Cancer Research

Michelle R. Huyser, Lyndsay A. Kandi, Agnes Premkumar, Kevin John Linn, Mackenzie Connon, Prince Andrew, and Nadine Caron

Abstract Indigenous people have experienced a combination of historical injustice, colonialism, and racism, which have resulted in health disparities. Data systems used to statistically quantify these inequities do not adequately account for these experiences and thus inadvertently impact meaningful use of this information to guide cancer treatment decisions and interventions in this patient population. To understand the Indigenous cancer experience, one must understand the inherent flaws in the data used to collect information about Indigenous people, the current

M. R. Huyser (✉)
University of Missouri, Department of Surgery, Surgical Oncology Division, Columbia, MO, USA
e-mail: mhuyser@health.missouri.edu

L. A. Kandi
Section of Plastic and Reconstructive Surgery, University of Chicago Medical Center, Chicago, IL, USA
e-mail: Lyndsay.Kandi@uchicagomedicine.org

A. Premkumar
Department of General Surgery, Creighton University School of Medicine, Phoenix, AZ, USA

K. J. Linn
Department of Global Health and Population, Harvard T.H. Chan School of Public Health, Boston, MA, USA

University of British Columbia, Vancouver, BC, Canada
e-mail: kevinlinn@hsph.harvard.edu

M. Connon
Northern Medical Program, University of British Columbia, Prince George, BC, Canada

P. Andrew
School of Population and Public Health, University of British Columbia, Vancouver, BC, Canada
e-mail: prince.andrew@ubc.ca

N. Caron
Centre for Excellence in Indigenous Health, Department of Surgery, University of British Columbia, Vancouver, BC, Canada

R. C. Haring (ed.), *Indigenous Genetics, Biobanking, Chemistry, and Cancer Research*, Cancer Health Disparities, https://doi.org/10.1007/978-3-032-17296-9_5

state of cancer in Indigenous people, and consider special circumstances in this patient population to guide the path forward in appropriate cancer care, especially surgical care. This chapter will demonstrate that Indigenous populations in the United States (US) (American Indian and Alaska Native—AI/AN) and Canada (First Nations, Metis, and Inuit) experience unique cancer journeys that require unique cancer solutions.

Definitions: where appropriate, the word Indigenous will be used pertaining to all Native communities from Canada and the US; however, when possible, distinctions-based terminology will be deployed when referring to findings that are specific to a community or group. In this case AI/AN when referring to Indigenous persons from the US and First Nations, Metis, and Inuit when referring to Indigenous persons from Canada.

Keywords Indigenous · American Indian/Alaska Native · First Nations · Metis · Inuit · Cancer · Surgery · Surgical oncology

1 Introduction

Cancer is a disease that affects all races, and for Indigenous people in the United States (US) and Canada. Understanding the profile of cancer outcomes is essential to ensuring equitable access to quality care and improving population outcomes. While advancements have been made in the detection, treatment, and survivorship of cancer, which have improved the cancer journey for many, including for Indigenous communities in North America, significant disparities in cancer outcomes persist. These disparities highlight that work is still needed from an equity perspective to improve cancer care service delivery for Indigenous people across the continent.

This chapter will demonstrate that Indigenous populations in the US (American Indian and Alaska Native—AI/AN) and Canada (First Nations, Metis, and Inuit) experience unique cancer journeys when accessing care compared to the general population and other racial groups. These disparities will be discussed and presented in this chapter with the recognition that these outcomes are often rooted in a combination of historical injustices, ongoing colonialism, systemic racism, and a lack of cultural safety within the healthcare system.

In the US, AI/AN populations are often categorized into six regions by the Indian Health Service (IHS), which provides 34% of the healthcare received by AI/AN populations and provides most of the information we know about the AI/AN patient population. The six regional categories include: Alaska, Pacific Coast, Northern Plains, Southern Plains, Southwest, and East (Wiggins et al., 2008). While AI/AN populations have the highest overall cancer incidence and mortality rates compared to all racial groups in the country, the incidence and prevalence of specific cancers vary significantly across the various regions and need to be considered in this context (Cancer, 2022).

In Canada, First Nations, Metis, and Inuit reflect significant heterogeneity culturally, linguistically, and world views. Despite these differences, recent studies have identified similarities in disparities in cancer outcomes across each population. In Canada, healthcare services are organized and delivered through Provinces and Territories, with Indigenous communities receiving most cancer care services through these publicly funded systems. This fragmentation hence presents challenges in forming a national picture of the Indigenous experience.

2 Cancer Data Challenges

When discussing cancer data within Indigenous populations, one must understand the limitations of the data forming the context of this information. The broad assessment of cancer among Indigenous populations in the US and Canada is fundamentally hampered by systematic data deficiencies. The underrepresentation and identification of Indigenous populations in cancer data is deeply rooted in a history of colonialism and exploitation, which has led to significant mistrust of research and data collection efforts within communities. Historically, Indigenous data was often collected without individual or community consent, exploiting communities under the guise of scientific inquiry (*Indigenous Data Sovereignty: Toward an agenda*, 2016). Such practices justified harmful policies by colonial governments, including forced displacement of communities from ancestral lands (Miller, 2019), and assimilationist policies like residential schools that intentionally dismantled Indigenous cultures by separating children from their families and suppressing their languages and traditions (Truth & Reconciliation Commission of, 2015). This legacy of control has instilled deep mistrust toward knowledge development activities from outside Indigenous communities.

These issues are evident in current data collection practices and the lack of Indigenous voices in shaping cancer research agendas, particularly in cancer surveillance. In the available large population databases, such as the Surveillance, Epidemiology, and End Results (SEER) program, AI/ANs are the most likely to be misclassified than any other race, leading to underreporting of cancer cases within these populations (Espey et al., 2014; Jim et al., 2014; Kruse et al., 2022). SEER relies on data sources such as death certificates, hospital records, and self-identification, all prone to errors in accurately capturing AI/AN identity (Espey et al., 2014). Many hospitals lack standardized methods for identifying AI/AN patients, and cultural competency gaps among healthcare staff further contribute to misclassification (Espey et al., 2014). Methods to reduce this misclassification in large databases includes utilizing classification ratios linked with Indian Health Service purchase/referred care delivery area counties but only reflects 34% of the AI/AN population (Jim et al., 2014; Kratzer et al., 2023). This misclassification also occurs on death certificates, leading to undercounting in cancer mortality and survival data statistics (Jim et al., 2014; Kratzer et al., 2023). Unfortunately, IHS linked cancer mortality is not publicly available in the same way that linked cancer incidence is publicly available, making efforts to reduce misclassification impossible (Cancer, 2022). Furthermore, AI/ANs populations are often listed as an "Other" group, merged into different ethnic data, or excluded completely from analyses.

The issue is compounded for urban Indigenous populations who reside off federally recognized tribal land, where approximately 71% of AI/AN individuals reside (Dignan et al., 2024). Many urban Indigenous people access healthcare through non-Indian Health Service (IHS) providers, where their Indigenous identity may not be recognized or adequately recorded. Moreover, medical systems outside of tribal healthcare facilities and the IHS are often not structured to accommodate the complexities of Indigenous identity, leading to further exclusion from cancer incidence data. Currently existing Indigenous life tables are thus not accurate nor reliable due to misclassification and numerator–denominator bias in vital statistics (Sarfati et al., 2018).

As a result of these data challenges, the effective planning and designing of health policies, programs, and services to meet the cancer care needs of Indigenous populations can be flawed. For instance, the perceived low rates of breast cancer among AI/AN women in the 1980s in the US sparked a debate over the necessity of screening mammography within the population. This debate led to policy decisions that deprioritized screening mammography services for early detection of breast cancer in AI/AN women (Frost et al., 1992). However, subsequent analyses revealed that after correcting for racial misclassification, breast cancer incidence rates among AI/AN women were twice as high as initially reported, highlighting significant gaps in cancer surveillance data (Frost et al., 1992). Similar issues exist with other cancer types, such as colorectal cancer, where underreporting and misclassification have hindered targeted screening initiatives. For example, Alaska Native communities have some of the highest colorectal cancer rates globally, but an initial lack of accurate data obscured this burden, delaying the implementation of widespread screening programs (Espey et al., 2014). Conversely, when accurate data are collected and utilized, they can lead to impactful policy changes. For example, the identification of higher-than-expected rates of lung cancer in Northern Plains AI/AN populations prompted regional tobacco cessation initiatives and increased funding for low-dose computed tomography (CT) screening programs in tribal communities (Dignan et al., 2024).

These examples demonstrate that a lack of reliable data not only skews health policy priorities but also exacerbates existing inequities, while accurate, culturally sensitive data collection can facilitate meaningful change. Addressing these deficiencies requires enhanced funding for Indigenous health research, improved classification practices in national registries, and active collaboration with AI/AN communities to ensure their voices and data sovereignty are respected (Espey et al., 2014; *Indigenous Data Sovereignty: Toward an agenda*, 2016). With these limitations in mind, we will now discuss current cancer trends by specific cancer type currently informing cancer treatment decisions with special consideration of surgical treatment when available.

3 Differences in Trends and Clinical Risk Factors by Specific Cancer

3.1 Cervical Cancer

Research from across US and Canadian jurisdictions finds that Indigenous women have significantly higher cervical cancer incidence rates than non-Indigenous women (Cancer, 2022; Decker et al., 2015; Jamal et al., 2021; Kratzer et al., 2023; Marrett & Chaudhry, 2003; Mazereeuw et al., 2018; Moore et al., 2015; Simkin et al., 2021). In British Columbia, cervical cancer is the fourth most diagnosed cancer, whereas it is the 12th most diagnosed cancer in non-First Nations women (McGahan et al., 2017). These findings are alarming, as cervical cancer is the fourth most diagnosed cancer globally, with most cases occurring in low- and middle-income countries with reduced access to preventative and screening services (Organization). Historically, in the US, screening rates among AI/ANs were less than 50% before government partnerships with tribal programs significantly increased these numbers (Buck DiSilvestro et al., 2024). In Canada, ongoing and intergenerational traumas have a major impact on Indigenous women's access to cervical cancer screening (Maar et al., 2013; Wakewich et al., 2016). One way to improve screening access for First Nations women is through culturally safe screening options. HPV self-screening is a preferred alternative to Pap smear for Indigenous communities globally and was well-received by 11 First Nations communities in Northwest Ontario (Styffe et al., 2019). First Nations women reported greater comfort and less fear and embarrassment with self-sampling than with the provider administered Pap smear (Wakewich et al., 2016; Zehbe et al., 2017). First Nations women also reported greater convenience, privacy, and control with self-sampling, ultimately empowering patients in the screening process (Wakewich et al., 2016; Zehbe et al., 2017). Beyond screening, access to culturally safe and effective cervical cancer treatment is needed and may be a barrier for First Nations women. Several studies have indicated that Indigenous women in Canada and the US diagnosed with cervical cancer experience higher mortality and poorer survival rates than non-Indigenous women (Kratzer et al., 2023; Louchini & Beaupré, 2008; Marrett & Chaudhry, 2003; Nishri et al., 2015).

3.2 Breast Cancer

Overall, breast cancer rates are lower among AI/AN populations compared to non-Hispanic Whites (NHWs) in the US, with incidence rates approximately 12–15% lower. However, there is notable regional variation among AI/ANs (Kratzer et al., 2023). For instance, in the US Southern Plains, the incidence of breast cancer is 35% higher than in NHWs in the same region, while the Southwest relative risk was significantly less than NHWs in the same region (Kratzer et al., 2023). These disparities can be attributed to several factors, including lower rates of cancer screening and limited access to medical care.

A national survey conducted between 2015 and 2018 revealed significant gaps in cancer screening, even among those utilizing IHS services. As expected, there is major variation between the regions and subregions for AI/AN mammography screening rates. These range from 45% to 70%, with only 52.0% of AI/AN women of screening age having had a screening mammogram in the two past years (Kratzer et al., 2023; Ward et al., 2004). In response, the Great Plains IHS implemented a mobile mammography unit from 2005 to 2017 to address transportation barriers. Additionally, the CDC's National Breast and Cervical Cancer Early Detection Program has partnered with tribal organizations to enhance screening and diagnostic services.

Breast cancer is a major health concern for Indigenous people in Canada as well. For example, the most common malignancy diagnosed in First Nations women in British Columbia is breast cancer, accounting for 34% of all cancers diagnosed (McGahan et al., 2017). In Ontario and Manitoba, First Nations women are diagnosed with breast cancer at later stages compared to non-First Nations women (Horrill et al., 2019; Sheppard et al., 2010). Organized population-based breast cancer screening programs are, therefore, important health system interventions. All Canadian jurisdictions have organized screening programs, except the territory of Nunavut (86% of the population self-report Indigenous identity in Nunavut—the largest being Inuit) (Cancer). However, despite the existence of these programs, participation in breast cancer screening is lower for Indigenous women. For example, it has been found that 37% of First Nations women in the province of Manitoba had a screening mammogram in the previous 2 years, from 1999 to 2008, compared to 59% of all other Manitoba women (Demers et al., 2015). In Nova Scotia, screening participation among First Nations women was consistently lower than all other Nova Scotia women in the 50–69 year age group (2004–2014), with only 36.5% of First Nations women screening in a recent period (2012–2014) (*Strength in Numbers Project*). These findings are concerning, as the Canadian performance target for screening participation is that at least 70% of women ages 50–69 years should be screened within a 30-month period.

In the US, AI/ANs experience three times longer travel times to all breast imaging modality facilities than all other racial groups (Onega et al., 2014). Additionally, AI/ANs with early-stage breast cancer are more likely to be treated with mastectomy than breast conserving therapy, while no surgical treatment differences have been demonstrated in later stages of breast cancer (Erdrich et al., 2022). Between AI/ANs and NHWs who received breast conserving therapy, AI/ANs were equally as likely to receive post lumpectomy radiation in early- and late-stage disease (Erdrich et al., 2022). However, AI/AN are twice as likely to receive partial breast irradiation than whole breast (Billar et al., 2014). Overall, AI/AN women are still less likely to receive guideline-based treatments like radiation or chemotherapy (Javid et al., 2014).

3.3 Colorectal Cancer

Colorectal cancer (CRC) screening is critical for AI/AN populations, especially since Alaska Natives have the highest CRC incidence rates in the world. Furthermore, AI/AN males are more likely to die from colorectal cancer compared to their NHW counterparts (Gopalani et al., 2020). Regionally, the incidence of CRC is particularly high in Alaska and the Northern Plains, where rates are double those in the Southwest (Kratzer et al., 2023). This disparity may be linked to dietary factors, such as higher consumption of sugar-sweetened beverages (Melkonian et al., 2021). While many AI/ANs are diagnosed at younger ages and later stages with CRC, CRC screening practices remain limited. In 2021, only 61.7% of AI/ANs had completed colorectal cancer screening when compared to 74.2% of NHW (Kratzer et al., 2023). In the Southwest, access to colorectal cancer screening is often restricted due to a lack of screening education and medical facilities with appropriate equipment. Many rely on fecal occult blood tests, with endoscopic options being extremely limited (Melkonian et al., 2019). This can be problematic, as AI/ANs have a large prevalence of *Helicobacter pylori*-related gastritis that can lead to false positive results from fecal occult blood tests (Kratzer et al., 2023). Despite these challenges, tribes have developed innovative screening programs like the Wisdom Steps program in the Northern Plains and Minnesota's Intertribal Colorectal Cancer Council as ways to improve screening and shift the paradigm of cancer care in these communities.

In Canada, incidence rates of CRC among both females and males between 1993 and 2010 were higher in First Nations males than non-First Nations (McGahan et al., 2017). Trends show increasing rates among First Nations females and males, while the incidence rates among non-First Nations have been decreasing for females and staying the same for males. CRC mortality is elevated in First Nations, especially in First Nations males. Incidence rate trends in First Nations and non-First Nations differed over the study period, causing a convergence or divergence in rates when comparing the two; however, one pattern noted was that First Nations incidence rates consistently increased over time (McGahan et al., 2017).

When undergoing surgical treatment for CRC, studies have conflicting findings. Some studies show AI/ANs are less likely to undergo colon resection while in other studies they are equally as likely to undergo colon resection for colon cancer (Markin et al., 2013; Nalluri et al., 2024; Ramkumar et al., 2022). Further exploration in this area is needed to clarify surgical treatment differences. Regarding adjuvant treatment, AI/ANs are less likely to receive adjuvant chemotherapy or adjuvant radiation therapy for CRC and are more likely to experience delay in initiation of adjuvant chemotherapy (Javid et al., 2014; Markin et al., 2013; Nalluri et al., 2024). Additionally, AI/ANs have poorer in-hospital mortality following rectal surgery compared to NHWs for unclear reasons (Markin et al., 2013).

3.4 Lung Cancer

Lung cancer incidence varies widely across AI/AN regions in the US. In the Southwest, the rate is approximately 16.8 cases per 100,000 compared to 109.3 cases per 100,000 in the Northern Plains (Kratzer et al., 2023). Unfortunately, lung cancer screening using low dose computed tomography (CT) scans is currently scarce among AI/AN populations. In places like BC, Canada, lung cancer screening with CT noncontrast scans only started in 2022 but efforts have begun trying to address geographic and cultural challenges for Indigenous Peoples in BC. The higher rates in the Northern and Southern Plains within the US are largely attributed to increased tobacco use in these regions, though it is essential to differentiate between traditional ceremonial tobacco use and commercial tobacco consumption. Previous studies have shown a correlation between higher commercial tobacco use and elevated cancer incidence in these regions (Melkonian et al., 2019).

Lung cancer is more often diagnosed at a younger age in AI/AN than NHWs (Schoephoerster et al., 2023). When diagnosed with lung cancer, AI/ANs are less likely to undergo surgical lung resection (Markin et al., 2013). When surgery is performed for early-stage cancer, AI/ANs are more likely to undergo wedge resection or nonsurgical management and less likely to undergo anatomic resection with lobectomy, bilobectomy, or pneumonectomy than NHWs (Schoephoerster et al., 2023). Some of this could be related to underlying lung function, but that information is not often available to correlate with surgical information in large databases. When AI/ANs are treated with anatomic resection at early lung cancer stages, they have similar outcomes as NHWs, but AI/ANs otherwise have a lower 5-year overall survival compared to NHWs (Schoephoerster et al., 2023).

3.5 Gastric Cancer

The incidence of gastric cancer is notably higher among AI/ANs compared to NHWs. ANs experience a rate four times higher, while AIs have a rate twice that of NHWs. In Canada, similar trends are seen with Indigenous communities in the Yukon and North West Territories having increased rates of gastric cancer (Colquhoun et al., 2019). For most people (49%) diagnosed with gastric cancer in the US, it is located in the proximal portion of the stomach, the cardia. Interestingly, most gastric cancers in AI/AN populations (48%) occur in the non-cardia portion of the stomach (Kratzer et al., 2023).

While the risk factors for cardia and non-cardia gastric cancers differ, both types are linked to cigarette smoking, which is more prevalent in AI/AN communities (Cancer, 2022). Cardia gastric cancer is also associated with obesity and gastroesophageal reflux disease (GERD). However, the prevalence of GERD in AI/AN populations has not been well-studied. In contrast, non-cardia gastric cancer is strongly associated with *Helicobacter pylori* infection, which is highly prevalent in

AI/AN populations, with an estimated prevalence of 75% among Alaskan Natives compared to 27% in the general population (Cancer, 2022; Kratzer et al., 2023). The prevalence of *H. pylori* is also higher in Indigenous communities in Yukon and North West Territories in Canada, with rates in communities between 58% and 69% compared to the non-Indigenous Canadian population. A primary risk factor for *H. pylori* infection is low socioeconomic status in both developing and developed countries. Other risk factors for *H. pylori* living rurally, water sanitation, smoking, alcohol consumption, crowded housing, and foods such as meat, raw milk, and vegetables (Bashir & Khan, 2023).

The survival rate for AI/AN individuals in the US with gastric cancer is 13% lower than for NHWs, with mortality rates 2.5 times higher between 2015 and 2019. This disparity is likely due to later diagnoses and differences in access to care. Fortunately, there has been some improvement in gastric cancer mortality rates among AI/AN populations from 1997 to 2019, and this trend is expected to continue (Kratzer et al., 2023). Similarly in Canada, mortality in northern Indigenous populations is increased in comparison to national averages.

When treated with surgery for gastric cancer, AI/ANs are more likely to have poor compliance to surgical treatment plans and start cancer treatment at later times compared to other races for unclear reasons (Liu et al., 2019). This likely contributes to AI/ANs having a poorer overall survival compared to NHWs (Rana et al., 2020). Largely little is known about surgical treatment in this patient population and needs more dedicated research.

3.6 Liver Cancer

AI/AN populations have the highest incidence of liver cancer compared to any other racial or ethnic group, with rates 2.5 times higher than those in NHWs (Kratzer et al., 2023). Key risk factors include obesity, type 2 diabetes, cigarette smoking, and chronic Hepatitis C infection. Individuals with chronic Hepatitis C are nearly 60 times more likely to develop hepatocellular carcinoma. Since 2019, the incidence of chronic Hepatitis C infection has been more than 2.5 times higher in AI/AN populations than in White individuals (Kratzer et al., 2023; Roubidoux et al., 2022). However, only 21% of the AI/AN population has been tested for Hepatitis C, suggesting a possible underreporting of true incidence rates (Roubidoux et al., 2022).

Access to treatment remains a major challenge, as antiviral medications are costly and often inaccessible to many in AI/AN communities. Despite these challenges, liver cancer in AI/AN populations is typically diagnosed at a similar stage to that in NHWs, and both groups have comparable 5-year relative survival rates (Roubidoux et al., 2022).

Hepatocellular carcinoma (HCC) overall survival ranges from 6 to 20 months following diagnosis (Golabi et al., 2017). Left untreated, patients with HCC have a 3.4 month median survival in advanced stage (Tian et al., 2020). Treatments include liver transplant, surgical resection, or locoregional liver-directed treatments with radiation, ablation, or arterial chemoembolization. Treatment decisions are based on patient underlying liver function, comorbidities, and patient preference. AI/ANs are diagnosed at younger ages (Xu et al., 2016), experience higher rates of hospitalization compared to other races ages 56–65, less likely to undergo surgical treatment with resection or liver transplant, and are more likely to be managed with ablation (Chikovsky et al., 2023; Xu et al., 2016; Yoshida et al., 2000). Some of this may be due to underlying liver dysfunction, as AI/ANs are more likely to present with cirrhosis at time of diagnosis (Xu et al., 2016). AI/ANs are also more likely to have in-hospital mortality compared to other races for unclear reasons (Chikovsky et al., 2023). These numbers are difficult to interpret, as correlation with surgical intervention and comorbidities are limited and further research is required.

3.7 *Kidney Cancer*

From 2014 to 2018, the incidence of kidney cancer among AI/AN individuals was 79% higher than that of NHWs (Kratzer et al., 2023). Major risk factors include obesity, cigarette smoking, kidney disease, hypertension, and diabetes. Obesity is particularly prevalent in AI/AN communities, due to factors such as limited access to nutritious foods and high consumption of sugar-sweetened beverages. AI/AN individuals also experience higher rates of type 2 diabetes than any other racial or ethnic group, which further contributes to the increased risk of kidney cancer (Kratzer et al., 2023). Between 2015 and 2019, the mortality rate for kidney cancer in AI/AN populations were 77% higher than for NHWs (Kratzer et al., 2023). Overall, AI/AN have higher incidence and mortality rates compared to NHWs (Gachupin et al., 2022). They are more likely to be diagnosed with clear cell renal cell carcinoma and at a younger age and most are diagnosed with grade 1 or grade 2 RCC than NHWs (Gachupin et al., 2022).

Compared to NHWs, AI/ANs are less likely to have any procedural treatment or undergo surgical nephrectomy (Gachupin et al., 2022). When undergoing nephrectomy, AI/ANs are more likely to undergo radical nephrectomy than partial nephrectomy compared to NHWs for unknown reasons (Gachupin et al., 2022). Similar to other cancers, little is known about surgical treatment in this patient population and requires more dedicated research.

4 Surgical Care

Currently, sparse information and few studies exist regarding surgical oncology care among Indigenous peoples. Thus, most studies about Indigenous cancer surgery are observational or retrospective from hospital systems with those patients. In the US, other studies involve large population data where numbers are too small for AI/AN people to be a significant number, so they are often left out completely or combined with other races. This is similar in the Canadian landscape, but two studies clearly document that with respect to overall surgical health services, Indigenous Peoples have lower access to surgical care, higher surgical complication rates and higher postoperative mortality rates (McVicar et al., 2021).

From the limited information we do have regarding surgical treatment of this patient population, Indigenous patients are more likely to undergo cancer surgery at rural hospitals in nonelective settings (Markin et al., 2013). AI/ANs are less likely to receive primary surgical therapy or undergo curative surgical resection or receive post-therapy surveillance across all cancer types (Javid et al., 2014). They are also more likely to have prolonged length of stay following surgery compared to other racial groups (Parsons et al., 2012). Further dedicated resources and research need to be invested in this area to explain these differences and how they may be impacting outcomes.

5 Special Surgical Considerations: Reconstruction Following Soft-Tissue Cancer Resection

Reconstructive surgery following oncologic resection, particularly postmastectomy breast reconstruction, is crucial in enhancing both physical and psychological outcomes. However, AI/AN populations experience significant disparities in accessing these services. The Women's Health and Cancer Rights Act (WHCRA) mandates insurance coverage for breast reconstruction following mastectomy; yet this policy does not extend to other reconstructive surgeries and remains inaccessible to many AI/AN individuals due to high rates of uninsurance and underinsurance (Kandi et al., 2025). Approximately 21% of AI/AN individuals are uninsured compared to 8% of the general US population, creating substantial barriers to both cancer treatment and reconstructive care (Warne & Frizzell, 2014).

Even when insurance is available, structural limitations within the Indian Health Service (IHS) exacerbate these disparities. With per capita spending at US$ 4078, less than half the amount allocated to Medicaid at US$ 8109, the IHS is unable to fund reconstructive surgeons or programs, forcing patients to seek care in external systems that often fail to align with cultural or logistical needs (Livermont et al., 2024). This systemic underfunding leaves IHS facilities without the capability to offer breast reconstruction, further marginalizing AI/AN women who already face elevated breast cancer mortality rates due to delayed diagnoses and limited access to cancer care (Jemal et al., 2004; Scott et al., 2024).

In theory, Canada does not have this insurance battle. For example, in BC, breast reconstruction is covered after mastectomy. However, access to plastic surgeons can be increasingly challenging as they are often not available in rural, northern communities where the other surgical breast cancer care can be provided. In BC, there are five geographic health authorities with the Northern Health authority comprising the northern two-thirds of the province (approximately 600,000 km^2 or 230,000 mi^2). In this vast geographic area, where there are 55 First Nations, there are only three plastic surgeons and all located at a single hospital in the southern border of the region.

Geographic barriers add another layer of inequity. AI/AN women frequently must travel three times longer than their non-Hispanic White counterparts to access reconstructive surgery, contributing to delays in care and lower utilization of reconstructive options (Ooi et al., 2011; Scott et al., 2024). A 2024 study highlighted that AI/AN women are 40% less likely to pursue breast reconstruction after mastectomy, a disparity attributed to logistical challenges, systemic inequities, and cultural factors, including perceptions that reconstruction is purely cosmetic and concerns over the use of acellular dermal matrices (Scott et al., 2024).

Cultural beliefs and preferences significantly influence decisions about reconstructive surgery. Many AI/AN women view breast reconstruction with autologous tissue as more culturally appropriate than implant-based methods and reject the use of tissue derived from deceased donors due to spiritual or cultural considerations (Scott et al., 2024). Additionally, low visibility of AI/AN needs in healthcare research and the misclassification of racial data further obscure the full extent of these disparities, hindering the development of targeted interventions (Gomez & Glaser, 2006; Kandi et al., 2025).

To address these systemic inequities, several steps must be taken. Increasing IHS funding specifically for reconstructive surgical services, expanding rural healthcare infrastructure, and fostering collaborations between tribal health systems and academic medical centers are essential. Moreover, culturally sensitive educational initiatives aimed at AI/AN communities could help alleviate misconceptions about reconstructive surgery. By adopting such measures, healthcare systems can work toward fulfilling the federal trust responsibilities to AI/AN populations, ensuring equitable access to reconstructive care (Kandi et al., 2025; Scott et al., 2024).

6 Cancer Genetics and Care: Evolving Uses, Historical Uses, Future Challenges

Like in breast reconstruction surgery, Indigenous cultural beliefs heavily inform cancer treatment decisions. As cancer treatment evolves and advances, these cultural beliefs may become more starkly evident. From a basic science perspective, cancer is a result of damage to genes from either defective genes, damage to genes from toxin exposure, or damage to genes from wearing out. Today genomic technology informs and guides cancer treatment toward tumor specific medicine. Whether patients know this or not, genomic testing of cancer cells are examined to determine how quickly cancer cells are likely to grow and inform what types of treatments may be helpful. Historically, cancer treatments were a one-size-fit-all approach according to the type of cancer by cell type. Now more genomic profiling of tumors has identified molecular targets that vary among the same cancer cell types in different individuals resulting in new therapies that can now target tumor specific markers. This has led to changes in sequencing treatments as well as an increasing role for surgery in metastatic settings. As tumor-directed medicine continues to be developed, it requires patients to participate in clinical trials where their tumors can be profiled to guide novel treatments. Genetic research among Indigenous communities remains highly contentious. DNA samples, among Indigenous communities, are considered sacred and part of a collective tribal group with religious and traditional significance (Garrison, 2013). Historically, the sacredness of this information has not always been respected by researchers working with these groups. Genetic information has been misused in highly charged topics including mental health, ethnic migration, and inbreeding often without the consent of the participants (Garrison, 2013). As a result, Indigenous communities are skeptical to participate in research trials and some communities have gone as far as to ban genetic research altogether (Freeman et al., 2021). Today less than 1% of genetic research includes AI/ANs (Barton et al., 2024). In order for additional molecular targets in cancer cells to be identified, research trials will need to continue to see if novel drugs are effective for different groups of people and types of cancers. If Indigenous people are left out of these trials, then vital information will be lost. Problematically, most Indigenous populations are in rural areas and may not have access to this tumor-directed advances since it requires access to facilities with access to molecular diagnostic laboratories. This also requires access to multidisciplinary teams, including radiation oncologists, medical oncologists, and surgical oncologists to discuss these cases and interpret findings to arrive at appropriate treatment regimens. Even if Indigenous patients can access tumor-directed therapy, these specific drugs may be cost prohibitive without additional financial assistance, so more will need to be done to overcome the barriers specific to this patient population.

7 Cancer Survival

As mentioned previously, interpreting cancer data in Indigenous patient populations requires cautious interpretation given database limitations and wide variation of statistical methods used to compare small group to larger population data (Nash et al., 2023). This is especially true when interpreting cancer survival data for Indigenous peoples. For example, when looking specifically at cancer survival rates if all-cause survival is used as the method to describe survival, then it needs to bear in mind that Indigenous populations tend to have a lower life expectancy, so all-cause mortality ratios will overestimate the disparity (Withrow et al., 2016). Furthermore, cause-specific survival may overestimate cancer survival in this population since death is linked to comorbidities rather than cancer, and Indigenous populations have a higher comorbidity index (Withrow et al., 2016). Despite this, utilizing cause-specific analysis can be helpful when population life expectancy tables are not accurate, as is the case in Indigenous populations (Nash et al., 2023). Using relative survival ratios as an alternative method also has its limitations since it relies on accurate population-specific estimates of mortality, which is not always accurate in Indigenous populations (Withrow et al., 2016). To adequately represent Indigenous cancer cases, multiple sources may need to be combined to capture more of these patients and prevent inadvertent bias, which requires concerted effort (Withrow et al., 2016). Thus, interpretation of survival analyses for Indigenous populations should be scrutinized to identify source of information, validity of the source, and limitations of the data source (Withrow et al., 2016). Hence, unique and innovative methods to elucidate this information from Indigenous populations will need to be developed in order to decolonize data.

In Canada, efforts have been underway to leverage linked data to understand cancer survival among Indigenous and non-Indigenous residents. For example, in British Columbia, research identified a concerning trend of lower survival across various cancer types (10 of 15 cancer sites examined in First Nations women and 10 of 12 cancer sites examined in First Nations men), with significantly lower survival seen for colorectal (men), kidney (men), non-Hodgkin lymphoma (men and women), and oral (men) and prostate cancer survival (McGahan et al., 2017). In Ontario, equally concerning are findings that show that less than half of First Nations people diagnosed with cancer survived 5 years following diagnosis compared to over half of non-First Nations people (Ontario). Yet these findings are not limited to First Nations, as it is also been found that for residents of Inuit Nunangat (the homeland of the Inuit), cancer is a major contributor to reduced life expectancy compared to the rest of Canada (Peters, 2010). These regional disparities underscore the need for a national perspective. Poorer access to care, including culturally safe care, may be an influential factor in these findings. In 2020, an independent investigation into Indigenous-specific racism and discrimination in the BC healthcare system confirmed that widespread racism exists within the system and that racism limits access to healthcare services. (Turpel-Lafond & Johnson, 2021). One way Canada is taking a federal approach to improving access to care is through the Canadian Strategy for Cancer Control, which includes First Nations, Inuit and Metis-specific actions (Cancer, 2019).

8 Conclusion

Up to this point, concentrated efforts in Indigenous cancer research has rightly focused on defining the scope of the problem through incidence and epidemiological cancer statistics. What we know from these efforts has highlighted inherent flaws in these data currently informing cancer treatment decision for Indigenous communities. As these methodologies improve, we must shift our efforts toward understanding current treatment trends and outcomes in these patient populations. Largely what we know about surgical cancer care in this patient population comes from retrospective or observational studies and large population databases representing only a small portion of the patient population and thus need to be interpreted with caution. Ultimately, to better understand surgical cancer care in this patient population, better methods to include Indigenous Peoples need to be devised and more dedicated research specific to this patient population is required. Once again, the paucity of access to cancer research funding and resources limits our understanding in this vital area of cancer care.

References

Barton, K. S., Porter, K. M., Mai, T., Claw, K. G., Hiratsuka, V. Y., Carroll, S. R., Burke, W., & Garrison, N. A. (2024). Genetic research within Indigenous communities: Engagement opportunities and pathways forward. *Genetics in Medicine, 26*(7), 101158. https://doi.org/10.1016/j.gim.2024.101158

Bashir, S., & Khan, M. (2023). Overview of Helicobacter pylori infection, prevalence, risk factors, and its prevention. *Advanced Gut & Microbiome Research, 2023*, 1–9. https://doi.org/10.1155/2023/9747027

Billar, J. A., Sim, M. S., & Chung, M. (2014). Increased use of partial-breast irradiation has not improved radiotherapy utilization for early-stage breast cancer. *Annals of Surgical Oncology, 21*(13), 4144–4151. https://doi.org/10.1245/s10434-014-3867-3

Buck DiSilvestro, J., Ulmer, K. K., Hedges, M., Kardonsky, K., & Bruegl, A. S. (2024). Cervical cancer: Preventable deaths among American Indian/Alaska Native Communities. *Obstetrics and Gynecology Clinics of North America, 51*(1), 125–141. https://doi.org/10.1016/j.ogc.2023.11.009

Cancer. (2022). *Special Section: Cancer in the American Indian and Alaska Native Population.* https://www.cancer.org/content/dam/cancer-org/research/cancer-facts-and-statistics/annual-cancer-facts-and-figures/2022/2022-special-section-aian.pdf

Cancer, C. P. A. (2019). *Canadian Strategy for Cancer Control.* https://s22457.pcdn.co/wp-content/uploads/2019/06/Canadian-Strategy-Cancer-Control-2019-2029 EN.pdf

Cancer, C. P. A. *Breast Cancer Screening in Canada.* https://www.partnershipagainstcancer.ca/topics/breast-cancer-screening-in-canada-2021-2022/programs/

Chikovsky, L., Kutuk, T., Rubens, M., Balda, A. N., Appel, H., Chuong, M. D., Kaiser, A., Hall, M. D., Contreras, J., Mehta, M. P., & Kotecha, R. (2023). Racial disparities in clinical presentation, surgical procedures, and hospital outcomes among patients with hepatocellular carcinoma in the United States. *Cancer Epidemiology, 82*, 102317. https://doi.org/10.1016/j.canep.2022.102317

Colquhoun, A., Hannah, H., Corriveau, A., Hanley, B., Yuan, Y., & Goodman, K. J. (2019). Gastric cancer in Northern Canadian populations: A focus on cardia and non-cardia subsites. *Cancers (Basel), 11*(4). https://doi.org/10.3390/cancers11040534

Decker, K. M., Demers, A. A., Kliewer, E. V., Biswanger, N., Musto, G., Elias, B., Griffith, J., & Turner, D. (2015). Pap test use and cervical cancer incidence in first nations women living in Manitoba. *Cancer Prevention Research, 8*(1), 49–55. https://doi.org/10.1158/1940-6207.Capr-14-0277

Demers, A. A., Decker, K. M., Kliewer, E. V., Musto, G., Shu, E., Biswanger, N., Fradette, K., Elias, B., Griffith, J., & Turner, D. (2015). Mammography rates for breast cancer screening: A comparison of First Nations women and all other women living in Manitoba, Canada, 1999-2008. *Preventing Chronic Disease, 12*, E82. https://doi.org/10.5888/pcd12.140571

Dignan, M. B., Burhansstipanov, L., Cina, K., Sargent, M., O'Connor, M., Tobacco, R., Ahamed, S. I., White, D. K., & Petereit, D. G. (2024). Low-dose computed tomography lung cancer screening for Northern Plains American Indians. In G. Garvey (Ed.), *Indigenous and tribal peoples and cancer* (pp. 197–201). Springer Nature. https://doi.org/10.1007/978-3-031-56806-0_41

Erdrich, J., Cordova-Marks, F., Monetathchi, A. R., Wu, M., White, A., & Melkonian, S. (2022). Disparities in breast-conserving therapy for non-Hispanic American Indian/Alaska native women compared with non-Hispanic White women. *Annals of Surgical Oncology, 29*(2), 1019–1030. https://doi.org/10.1245/s10434-021-10730-7

Espey, D. K., Jim, M. A., Cobb, N., Bartholomew, M., Becker, T., Haverkamp, D., & Plescia, M. (2014). Leading causes of death and all-cause mortality in American Indians and Alaska Natives. *American Journal of Public Health, 104 Suppl 3*(Suppl 3), S303–S311. https://doi.org/10.2105/AJPH.2013.301798

Freeman, A. A., Arbuckle, J., & Petty, E. M. (2021). Preparing genetic counselors to serve Native American communities. *Journal of Genetic Counseling, 30*(5), 1388–1398. https://doi.org/10.1002/jgc4.1405

Frost, F., Taylor, V., & Fries, E. (1992). Racial misclassification of Native Americans in a surveillance, epidemiology, and end results cancer registry. *Journal of the National Cancer Institute, 84*(12), 957–962. https://doi.org/10.1093/jnci/84.12.957

Gachupin, F. C., Lee, B. R., Chipollini, J., Pulling, K. R., Cruz, A., Wong, A. C., Valencia, C. I., Hsu, C. H., & Batai, K. (2022). Renal cell carcinoma surgical treatment disparities in American Indian/Alaska Natives and Hispanic Americans in Arizona. *International Journal of Environmental Research and Public Health, 19*(3). https://doi.org/10.3390/ijerph19031185

Garrison, N. A. (2013). Genomic justice for Native Americans: Impact of the Havasupai case on genetic research. *Science, Technology, & Human Values, 38*(2), 201–223. https://doi.org/10.1177/0162243912470009

Golabi, P., Fazel, S., Otgonsuren, M., Sayiner, M., Locklear, C. T., & Younossi, Z. M. (2017). Mortality assessment of patients with hepatocellular carcinoma according to underlying disease and treatment modalities. *Medicine (Baltimore), 96*(9), e5904. https://doi.org/10.1097/MD.0000000000005904

Gomez, S. L., & Glaser, S. L. (2006). Misclassification of race/ethnicity in a population-based cancer registry (United States). *Cancer Causes & Control, 17*(6), 771–781. https://doi.org/10.1007/s10552-006-0013-y

Gopalani, S. V., Janitz, A. E., Martinez, S. A., Gutman, P., Khan, S., & Campbell, J. E. (2020). Trends in cancer incidence among American Indians and Alaska Natives and non-Hispanic Whites in the United States, 1999-2015. *Epidemiology, 31*(2), 205–213. https://doi.org/10.1097/EDE.0000000000001140

Horrill, T. C., Dahl, L., Sanderson, E., Munro, G., Garson, C., Fransoo, R., Thompson, G., Cook, C., Linton, J., & Schultz, A. S. H. (2019). Cancer incidence, stage at diagnosis and outcomes among Manitoba First Nations people living on and off reserve: A retrospective population-based analysis. *CMAJ Open, 7*(4), E754–e760. https://doi.org/10.9778/cmajo.20190176

Indigenous Data Sovereignty: Toward an agenda. (2016). (Vol. 38). ANU Press. http://www.jstor.org/stable/j.ctt1q1crgf

Jamal, S., Jones, C., Walker, J., Mazereeuw, M., Sheppard, A. J., Henry, D., & Marrett, L. D. (2021). Cancer in First Nations people in Ontario, Canada: Incidence and mortality, 1991 to 2010. *Health Reports, 32*(6), 14–28. https://doi.org/10.25318/82-003-x202100600002-eng

Javid, S. H., Varghese, T. K., Morris, A. M., Porter, M. P., He, H., Buchwald, D., Flum, D. R., & Collaborative to Improve Native Cancer, O. (2014). Guideline-concordant cancer care and survival among American Indian/Alaskan Native patients. *Cancer, 120*(14), 2183–2190. https://doi.org/10.1002/cncr.28683

Jemal, A., Clegg, L. X., Ward, E., Ries, L. A., Wu, X., Jamison, P. M., Wingo, P. A., Howe, H. L., Anderson, R. N., & Edwards, B. K. (2004). Annual report to the nation on the status of cancer, 1975-2001, with a special feature regarding survival. *Cancer, 101*(1), 3–27. https://doi.org/10.1002/cncr.20288

Jim, M. A., Arias, E., Seneca, D. S., Hoopes, M. J., Jim, C. C., Johnson, N. J., & Wiggins, C. L. (2014). Racial misclassification of American Indians and Alaska Natives by Indian Health Service Contract Health Service Delivery Area. *American Journal of Public Health, 104 Suppl 3*(Suppl 3), S295–S302. https://doi.org/10.2105/AJPH.2014.301933

Kandi, L. A., Livermont, T. E., & Weaver, T. L. (2025). Disparities in postmastectomy reconstruction use among American Indian and Alaska Native women. *Plastic and Reconstructive Surgery, 155*(3), 642e–643e. https://doi.org/10.1097/PRS.0000000000011730

Kratzer, T. B., Jemal, A., Miller, K. D., Nash, S., Wiggins, C., Redwood, D., Smith, R., & Siegel, R. L. (2023). Cancer statistics for American Indian and Alaska Native individuals, 2022: Including increasing disparities in early onset colorectal cancer. *CA: a Cancer Journal for Clinicians, 73*(2), 120–146. https://doi.org/10.3322/caac.21757

Kruse, G., Lopez-Carmen, V. A., Jensen, A., Hardie, L., & Sequist, T. D. (2022). The Indian Health Service and American Indian/Alaska Native health outcomes. *Annual Review of Public Health, 43*, 559–576. https://doi.org/10.1146/annurev-publhealth-052620-103633

Liu, G., Xu, M., Gao, T., Xu, L., Zeng, P., Bo, H., Li, F., Zhang, W., & Wang, Z. (2019). Surgical compliance and outcomes in gastric cancer: A population-based cohort study. *Journal of Cancer, 10*(4), 779–788. https://doi.org/10.7150/jca.29073

Livermont, T. E., Kandi, L. A., & Weaver, T. L. (2024). Invisibility of Native American communities in plastic and reconstructive surgery: The role of tribal sovereignty and self-governance to improve access. *Plastic and Reconstructive Surgery. Global Open, 12*(9), e6177. https://doi.org/10.1097/GOX.0000000000006177

Louchini, R., & Beaupré, M. (2008). Cancer incidence and mortality among Aboriginal people living on reserves and northern villages in Quebec, 1988-2004. *International Journal of Circumpolar Health, 67*(5), 445–451. https://doi.org/10.3402/ijch.v67i5.18355

Maar, M., Burchell, A., Little, J., Ogilvie, G., Severini, A., Yang, J., & Zehbe, I. (2013). A qualitative study of provider perspectives of structural barriers to cervical cancer screening among first nations women. *Women's Health Issues, 23*(5), e319–e325. https://doi.org/10.1016/j.whi.2013.06.005

Markin, A., Habermann, E. B., Zhu, Y., Abraham, A., Ahluwalia, J. S., Vickers, S. M., & Al-Refaie, W. B. (2013). Cancer surgery among American Indians. *JAMA Surgery, 148*(3), 277-284; discussion 284. https://doi.org/10.1001/jamasurg.2013.1423

Marrett, L. D., & Chaudhry, M. (2003). Cancer incidence and mortality in Ontario First Nations, 1968-1991 (Canada). *Cancer Causes & Control, 14*(3), 259–268. https://doi.org/10.1023/a:1023632518568

Mazereeuw, M. V., Withrow, D. R., Diane Nishri, E., Tjepkema, M., & Marrett, L. D. (2018). Cancer incidence among First Nations adults in Canada: Follow-up of the 1991 Census Mortality Cohort (1992-2009). *Canadian Journal of Public Health, 109*(5–6), 700–709. https://doi.org/10.17269/s41997-018-0091-0

McGahan, C. E., Linn, K., Guno, P., Johnson, H., Coldman, A. J., Spinelli, J. J., & Caron, N. R. (2017). Cancer in First Nations people living in British Columbia, Canada: An analysis of incidence and survival from 1993 to 2010. *Cancer Causes & Control, 28*(10), 1105–1116. https://doi.org/10.1007/s10552-017-0950-7

McVicar, J. A., Poon, A., Caron, N. R., Bould, M. D., Nickerson, J. W., Ahmad, N., Kimmaliardjuk, D. M., Sheffield, C., Champion, C., & McIsaac, D. I. (2021). Postoperative outcomes for indigenous peoples in Canada: A systematic review. *CMAJ, 193*(20), E713–e722. https://doi.org/10.1503/cmaj.191682

Melkonian, S. C., Jim, M. A., Haverkamp, D., Wiggins, C. L., McCollum, J., White, M. C., Kaur, J. S., & Espey, D. K. (2019). Disparities in cancer incidence and trends among American Indians and Alaska Natives in the United States, 2010-2015. *Cancer Epidemiology, Biomarkers & Prevention, 28*(10), 1604–1611. https://doi.org/10.1158/1055-9965.EPI-19-0288

Melkonian, S. C., Weir, H. K., Jim, M. A., Preikschat, B., Haverkamp, D., & White, M. C. (2021). Incidence of and trends in the leading cancers with elevated incidence among American Indian and Alaska Native populations, 2012-2016. *American Journal of Epidemiology, 190*(4), 528–538. https://doi.org/10.1093/aje/kwaa222

Miller, R. J. (2019). THE DOCTRINE OF DISCOVERY The International Law of Colonialism. *The Indigenous Peoples' Journal of Law, Culture, & Resistance, 5*, 35–42. https://www.jstor.org/stable/48671863

Moore, S. P., Antoni, S., Colquhoun, A., Healy, B., Ellison-Loschmann, L., Potter, J. D., Garvey, G., & Bray, F. (2015). Cancer incidence in indigenous people in Australia, New Zealand, Canada, and the USA: A comparative population-based study. *The Lancet Oncology, 16*(15), 1483–1492. https://doi.org/10.1016/s1470-2045(15)00232-6

Nalluri, H., Marmor, S., Prathibha, S., Jenkins, A., Dindinger-Hill, K., Kihara, M., Sundberg, M. A., Day, L. W., Owen, M. J., Lowry, A. C., & Tuttle, T. M. (2024). Evaluating disparities in Colon cancer survival in American Indian/Alaskan native patients using the National Cancer Database. *Journal of Racial and Ethnic Health Disparities, 11*(4), 2407–2415. https://doi.org/10.1007/s40615-023-01706-2

Nash, S. H., Wahlen, M. M., Meisner, A. L. W., & Morawski, B. M. (2023). Choice of survival metric and its impacts on cancer survival estimates for American Indian and Alaska Native people. *Cancer Epidemiology, Biomarkers & Prevention, 32*(3), 398–405. https://doi.org/10.1158/1055-9965.EPI-22-1059

Nishri, E. D., Sheppard, A. J., Withrow, D. R., & Marrett, L. D. (2015). Cancer survival among First Nations people of Ontario, Canada (1968-2007). *International Journal of Cancer, 136*(3), 639–645. https://doi.org/10.1002/ijc.29024

Onega, T., Hubbard, R., Hill, D., Lee, C. I., Haas, J. S., Carlos, H. A., Alford-Teaster, J., Bogart, A., DeMartini, W. B., Kerlikowske, K., Virnig, B. A., Buist, D. S., Henderson, L., & Tosteson, A. N. (2014). Geographic access to breast imaging for US women. *Journal of the American College of Radiology, 11*(9), 874–882. https://doi.org/10.1016/j.jacr.2014.03.022

Ontario, C. C. *Cancer in First Nations people in Ontario: Incidence, mortality, survival and prevalence.* https://www.cancercareontario.ca/en/statistical-reports/cancer-first-nations-people-ontario-incidence-mortality-survival-and-prevalence#:~:text=Less%20than%20half%20of%20First,(60%20percent)%20in%20Ontario

Ooi, S. L., Martinez, M. E., & Li, C. I. (2011). Disparities in breast cancer characteristics and outcomes by race/ethnicity. *Breast Cancer Research and Treatment, 127*(3), 729–738. https://doi.org/10.1007/s10549-010-1191-6

Organization, W. H. *Cervical Cancer.* https://www.who.int/news-room/fact-sheets/detail/cervical-cancer

Parsons, H. M., Habermann, E. B., Stain, S. C., Vickers, S. M., & Al-Refaie, W. B. (2012). What happens to racial and ethnic minorities after cancer surgery at American College of Surgeons National Surgical Quality Improvement Program hospitals? *Journal of the American College of Surgeons, 214*(4), 539–547; discussion 547–539. https://doi.org/10.1016/j.jamcollsurg.2011.12.024

Peters, P. A. (2010). Causes and contributions to differences in life expectancy for Inuit Nunangat and Canada, 1994-2003. *International Journal of Circumpolar Health, 69*(1), 38–49. https://doi.org/10.3402/ijch.v69i1.17429

Ramkumar, N., Colla, C. H., Wang, Q., O'Malley, A. J., Wong, S. L., & Brooks, G. A. (2022). Association of rurality, race and ethnicity, and socioeconomic status with the surgical management of Colon cancer and postoperative outcomes among medicare beneficiaries. *JAMA Network Open, 5*(8), e2229247. https://doi.org/10.1001/jamanetworkopen.2022.29247

Rana, N., Gosain, R., Lemini, R., Wang, C., Gabriel, E., Mohammed, T., Siromoni, B., & Mukherjee, S. (2020). Socio-demographic disparities in gastric adenocarcinoma: A population-based study. *Cancers (Basel), 12*(1). https://doi.org/10.3390/cancers12010157

Roubidoux, M. A., Kaur, J. S., & Rhoades, D. A. (2022). Health disparities in cancer among American Indians and Alaska Natives. *Academic Radiology, 29*(7), 1013–1021. https://doi.org/10.1016/j.acra.2021.10.011

Sarfati, D., Garvey, G., Robson, B., Moore, S., Cunningham, R., Withrow, D., Griffiths, K., Caron, N. R., & Bray, F. (2018). Measuring cancer in indigenous populations. *Annals of Epidemiology, 28*(5), 335–342. https://doi.org/10.1016/j.annepidem.2018.02.005

Schoephoerster, J., Praska, C., White, M., Salami, A., Marmor, S., Andrade, R., Bhargava, A., Diaz-Gutierrez, I., Hui, J., Tuttle, T., Owen, M., & Rao, M. (2023). A nationwide analysis of disparities in guideline-concordant care in American Indians and Alaska Natives with stage I non-small cell lung cancer. *Journal of Thoracic Disease, 15*(11), 5891–5900. https://doi.org/10.21037/jtd-23-801

Scott, K., Marquez, J., Tausinga, T., & Tuncer, F. (2024). Attitudes toward breast reconstruction among American Indian/Alaska Native women in the Mountain West Region: A qualitative study. *Plastic and Reconstructive Surgery – Global Open, 12*(1S2), 8–9. https://doi.org/10.1097/01.GOX.0001010356.95754.e9

Sheppard, A. J., Chiarelli, A. M., Marrett, L. D., Mirea, L., Nishri, E. D., & Trudeau, M. E. (2010). Detection of later stage breast cancer in First Nations women in Ontario, Canada. *Canadian Journal of Public Health, 101*(1), 101–105. https://doi.org/10.1007/bf03405573

Simkin, J., Smith, L., van Niekerk, D., Caird, H., Dearden, T., van der Hoek, K., Caron, N. R., Woods, R. R., Peacock, S., & Ogilvie, G. (2021). Sociodemographic characteristics of women with invasive cervical cancer in British Columbia, 2004-2013: A descriptive study. *CMAJ Open, 9*(2), E424–e432. https://doi.org/10.9778/cmajo.20200139

Strength in Numbers Project. http://www.tuikn.ca/wp-content/uploads/2015/03/cancer_print_proof_final-1.pdf

Styffe, C., Tratt, E., Macdonald, M., & Brassard, P. (2019). HPV self-sampling in indigenous communities: A scoping review. *Journal of Immigrant and Minority Health, 22*(4), 852–859. https://doi.org/10.1007/s10903-019-00954-x

Tian, H., Cao, S., Hu, M., Wang, Y., Fu, Q., Pan, Y., & Qin, T. (2020). Identification of predictive factors in hepatocellular carcinoma outcome: A longitudinal study. *Oncology Letters, 20*(1), 765–773. https://doi.org/10.3892/ol.2020.11581

Truth, & Reconciliation Commission of, C. (2015). *Canada's Residential Schools: The History, part 1, origins to 1939 the final report of the Truth and Reconciliation Commission of Canada, Volume I*. McGill-Queen's University Press. https://doi.org/10.2307/j.ctt19rm9v4.

Turpel-Lafond, L.-F., & Johnson. (2021). In Plain Sight: Elaboration on the review. *BC Medical Journal, 63*(2), 83–88.

Wakewich, P., Wood, B., Davey, C., Laframboise, A., & Zehbe, I. (2016). Colonial legacy and the experience of First Nations women in cervical cancer screening: A Canadian multi-community study. *Critical Public Health, 26*(4), 368–380. https://doi.org/10.1080/09581596.2015.1067671

Ward, E., Jemal, A., Cokkinides, V., Singh, G. K., Cardinez, C., Ghafoor, A., & Thun, M. (2004). Cancer disparities by race/ethnicity and socioeconomic status. *CA: a Cancer Journal for Clinicians, 54*(2), 78–93. https://doi.org/10.3322/canjclin.54.2.78

Warne, D., & Frizzell, L. B. (2014). American Indian health policy: Historical trends and contemporary issues. *American Journal of Public Health, 104 Suppl 3*(Suppl 3), S263–S267. https://doi.org/10.2105/AJPH.2013.301682

Wiggins, C. L., Espey, D. K., Wingo, P. A., Kaur, J. S., Wilson, R. T., Swan, J., Miller, B. A., Jim, M. A., Kelly, J. J., & Lanier, A. P. (2008). Cancer among American Indians and Alaska Natives in the United States, 1999-2004. *Cancer, 113*(5 Suppl), 1142–1152. https://doi.org/10.1002/cncr.23734

Withrow, D. R., Racey, C. S., & Jamal, S. (2016). A critical review of methods for assessing cancer survival disparities in Indigenous population. *Annals of Epidemiology, 26*(8), 579–591. https://doi.org/10.1016/j.annepidem.2016.06.007

Xu, L., Kim, Y., Spolverato, G., Gani, F., & Pawlik, T. M. (2016). Racial disparities in treatment and survival of patients with hepatocellular carcinoma in the United States. *Hepatobiliary Surgery and Nutrition, 5*(1), 43–52. https://doi.org/10.3978/j.issn.2304-3881.2015.08.05

Yoshida, E. M., Caron, N. R., Buczkowski, A. K., Arbour, L. T., Scudamore, C. H., Steinbrecher, U. P., Erb, S. R., & Chung, S. W. (2000). Indications for liver transplantation in British Columbia's Aboriginal population: A 10-year retrospective analysis. *Canadian Journal of Gastroenterology, 14*(9), 775–779. https://doi.org/10.1155/2000/907463

Zehbe, I., Wakewich, P., King, A. D., Morrisseau, K., & Tuck, C. (2017). Self-administered versus provider-directed sampling in the Anishinaabek Cervical Cancer Screening Study (ACCSS): A qualitative investigation with Canadian First Nations women. *BMJ Open, 7*(8), e017384. https://doi.org/10.1136/bmjopen-2017-017384

2020 Population Updates for Cancer Mortality: An Oklahoma, USA, Experience

Janis E. Campbell, Mark P. Doescher, Amanda E. Janitz, Del V. Beaver, and Lancer D. Stephens

Abstract This chapter examines the impact of the 2020 US Census policy changes on age-adjusted cancer mortality rates among American Indian and Alaska Native (AIAN) populations in Oklahoma. Historically, the US Census used "bridged" population estimates to align multiracial respondents with pre-2000 racial categories. With the 2020 Census, this approach was discontinued, shifting to a six-race classification, significantly affecting AIAN population estimates. Given that AIAN populations have some of the highest documented cancer mortality rates, particularly in the Southern Plains, Northern Plains, and Alaska, this change raises concerns about the accuracy of cancer burden assessments.

This chapter analyzes Oklahoma's AIAN cancer mortality trends using Oklahoma Vital Statistics and the OK2SHARE public health database. By comparing mortality rates under the four-race bridged and six-race estimates, the study highlights

J. E. Campbell (✉)
Department of Biostatistics and Epidemiology, The University of Oklahoma Health Campus, Oklahoma City, OK, USA

Stephenson Cancer Center, The University of Oklahoma Health Campus, Oklahoma City, OK, USA
e-mail: Janis-Campbell@ou.edu

M. P. Doescher
Stephenson Cancer Center, The University of Oklahoma Health Campus, Oklahoma City, OK, USA
e-mail: Mark-Doescher@ou.edu

A. E. Janitz
Department of Biostatistics and Epidemiology, The University of Oklahoma Health Campus, Oklahoma City, OK, USA
e-mail: Amanda-Janitz@ou.edu

D. V. Beaver
The Muscogee Nation, Muscogee Reservation, Okmulgee, OK, USA

L. D. Stephens
Oklahoma Shared Clinical and Translational Resources, The University of Oklahoma Health Campus, Oklahoma City, OK, USA
e-mail: Lancer-Stephens@ou.edu

R. C. Haring (ed.), *Indigenous Genetics, Biobanking, Chemistry, and Cancer Research*, Cancer Health Disparities, https://doi.org/10.1007/978-3-032-17296-9_6

change not due to screening or healthcare access but to revised population denominators. Findings show a statistically significant decrease in AIAN cancer mortality rates under the six-race system, likely due to shifts in racial categorization. The results highlight the sociopolitical nature of racial classification and its implications for the interpretation of public health data. This chapter aims to inform non-epidemiologists, including policymakers and journalists, about the complexities of racial data reporting and its real-world consequences.

Keywords US Census · Cancer mortality · American Indian or Alaska Native · Health disparities · Race

Abbreviations

AIAN	American Indian or Alaska Native
AAMR	Age-adjusted Mortality Rate
ACOG	Association of Central Oklahoma Governments
ASCOG	Association of South Central Oklahoma Governments
COEDD	Central Oklahoma Economic Development District
EODD	Eastern Oklahoma Development District
GGEDA	Grand Gateway Economic Development Association
INCOG	Indian Nations Council of Governments
ITU	Indian Health Services/Tribal Health Services/Urban Indian Clinics
KEDDO	Kiamichi Economic Development District of Oklahoma
NODA	Northern Oklahoma Development Authority
OEDA	Oklahoma Economic Development Authority
OK2SHARE	**Ok**lahoma **S**tatistics on **H**ealth **A**vailable fo**r** **E**veryone
OVS	Oklahoma Vital Statistics
RR	Rate Ratio
SODA	Southern Oklahoma Development Association
SSPD	Substate Planning Districts
SWODA	South Western Oklahoma Developmental Authority
US	United States

1 Introduction

Every 10 years in the United States (US), new census data necessitates adjustments to mortality rates. These new 10-year census estimates are often dramatically different from previous estimates, with increases in the distribution of populations by age, race, ethnicity, and geographic location being common (Frey, 2021). With the adoption of the American Community Survey in 2005, census differences became less dramatic as it allowed for more accurate intercensal estimates (United States Census Bureau, 2017). It has been established that these denominator changes can significantly adjust morbidity and mortality rates (Amodio et al., 2021; Rhee & Klompas, 2020). Starting in 2000, the US Census began using "bridged" population estimates (Allen & Turner, 2001; Ingram et al., 2003; Parker et al., 2004; Statistics, 2003). The bridged population estimates utilized National Health Interview Survey responses and contextual county-level information to develop models that bridged multiracial respondents to the pre-2000 single-race census racial categories (Allen & Turner, 2001; Ingram et al., 2003; Parker et al., 2004; Statistics, 2003). These bridged estimates have been used for the last 20 years. With the release of the 2020 census estimates, some institutions have discontinued using the bridged-race population estimates. Although the change was planned, it had an unintended but significant impact on American Indian and Alaska Native (AIAN) population data (Ingram et al., 2003; Parker et al., 2004; White et al., 2014b).

Historically and currently, there have been issues with the misclassification of AIAN people across various research and clinical practice databases (Haozous et al., 2014; Layne et al., 2019). The implications are far-reaching, as misclassification can distort reported cancer rates of the AIAN population. This is an issue of numerator and denominator dissonance. The most common solution to the dissonance between the numerator and denominator has been to update the numerator using a linking process with Indian Health Services, Tribal Health Services, and Urban Indian Clinics (I/T/U) data (Kunitz et al., 2014; Li et al., 2014; Llaneza et al., 2024; Plescia et al., 2014; Singh et al., 2014; White et al., 2014a, b). An additional solution has been to link to tribal rolls (Haring et al., 2018; Michalek et al., 1989; Stehr-Green et al., 2002; Yankaskas et al., 2009), which is a more accurate process. Many Tribal Nations, however, will not allow their rolls to be used in such research due to historical abuse of research or a lack of capacity. Revised estimates using the bridged denominator and enhanced numerator from linkages with I/T/U data are arguably the most accurate estimates of the true cancer burden among the AIAN population.

When analyses account for misclassification, the AIAN population has had some of the highest documented age-adjusted cancer mortality rates in the US, particularly in the Southern Plains, Northern Plains, and Alaska (Espey et al., 2014a; Hoffman et al., 2014). For some cancers, the incidence rates were also very high (Espey et al., 2014a; Kills First et al., 2022; Kratzer et al., 2022; Melkonian et al., 2022; Wiggins et al., 2008a).

With the release of the 2020 census, the denominator has changed due to the implementation of new policies for categorizing the data. The data no longer uses bridged population estimates, but recognizes a multi-race population (up to five racial groups) as a racial category. For this chapter, we are interested in documenting changes in the age-adjusted mortality rate in Oklahoma before and after the implementation of this change. We chose Oklahoma for three reasons. First, Oklahoma has a large AIAN population, second only to California when considering AIAN race alone. Second, Oklahoma has Oklahoma Statistics on Health

Available for Everyone (OK2SHARE), a web-based query system using public health datasets (https://www.health.state.ok.us/). This system enables the use of de-identified data with both methods for the same years. Using Oklahoma data provides some insight into the impact of these changes on the AIAN cancer mortality rate. Third, Oklahoma has a significant multiracial population, with 12.8% of the population reporting two or more races on the 2020 census. This chapter aims to describe the changing AIAN mortality rates based on population estimates for the 2020 population revision and policy changes. The objective is to provide an understanding of these changing rates.

2 Methods

2.1 Data Sources

This chapter used age-adjusted cancer mortality rates standardized to the 2000 US Census population. Mortality rates were presented for all cancer sites combined and for the most common 32 cancer causes of death among the AIAN populations; site categories were consistent with prevailing reporting standards. Lymphomas (ICD-O histology codes 9590–9729) were presented as separate categories (i.e., Hodgkin and non-Hodgkin lymphoma). Mesothelioma (ICD-O histology codes 9050–9055) and Kaposi sarcoma (ICD-O-3 histology code 9140) were excluded from the analysis with other tumors of specific anatomic sites. In situ and invasive bladder tumors were combined into a single category. All other benign and tumors of uncertain, borderline, or low malignant potential (ICD-O-3 behavior codes 0 and 2, respectively) were excluded from the analysis, as were tumors of uncertain or unknown behavior (ICD-O-3 behavior code 9). Cancer mortality data for 2016–2020 were obtained from the Oklahoma Vital Statistics (OVS). OVS is a surveillance system designed and implemented to collect all deaths in Oklahoma. All data sources were publicly available through OK2SHARE, a web-based query system that enables analysis of public health datasets (https://www.health.state.ok.us/). For trend data, 2010 was the first-year of data available for Oklahoma, as multiracial categories became available on death certificates.

2.2 Racial Categories

This chapter used the term AIAN to describe the Indigenous population of the US, as it is the official US Census terminology for race. It is essential to note that AIAN populations have historically been, and continue to be, mistakenly classified as a race for data collection purposes. In reality, AIAN populations constitute hundreds of Tribal Nations with congressionally deemed federal recognition. As of January 30, 2026, there are 575 federally recognized Tribes listed on the Federal Register notice. Thus, each of the current Tribes within the US is not a racial group, but rather a governmental and political entity, each with a sovereign Tribal government-to-US government relationship. However, given the current data-gathering processes that identified AIAN as a race, this chapter will continue to focus on provided race-based data (including AIAN) and the importance of race-based mortality estimates.

This chapter begins with a comparison of different population estimates and age-adjusted mortality rates for populations by race in Oklahoma. The bridged race estimates (four-race group) included White, Black, AIAN, and Asian. Updated (six-race group) categories included White, Black, AIAN, Asian, Native Hawaiian and Pacific Islander, and two or more races. Hispanic origin did not change. Moreover, the Census Bureau made a policy change in how it determined multi-race. If someone reported being Black or White, they were asked about their origins. If their origins were from a region not classified as the same race by Census Bureau policy, they were listed as multi-race with another race as their second racial group (Starr & Pao, 2024). These individuals only chose one race but were recoded to multiracial, sometimes inappropriately (Starr & Pao, 2024).

2.3 *Geography*

For geographic analysis, substate planning districts were used. Substate planning districts (SSPD) are voluntary associations of local governments. They address problems and planning needs that transcend the boundaries of individual local governments. Substate planning districts, for example, complete regional data collection and analysis, mapping, and coordination of environmental, economic, and social program plans, as well as rural fire defense, capital improvements planning, and emergency response planning. There are 11 substate planning districts in Oklahoma, each encompassing between three counties and 10 counties. (Fig. 1). The planning districts are: ACOG-Association of Central Oklahoma Governments, ASCOG-Association of South Central Oklahoma Governments, COEDD-Central Oklahoma Economic Development District, EODD-Eastern Oklahoma Development District, GGEDA-Grand Gateway Economic Development Association, INCOG-Indian Nations Council of Governments, KEDDO-Kiamichi Economic Development District of Oklahoma, NODA-Northern Oklahoma Development Authority, OEDA-Oklahoma Economic Development Authority, SODA-Southern Oklahoma Development Association, and SWODA-Southwestern Oklahoma Developmental Authority.

2.4 *Statistical Analysis*

Using age-adjusted mortality rates standardized to the 2000 US population, age-adjusted mortality rate ratios (RRs) were computed for the four-race bridged and six-race estimates. Rates were omitted if there were fewer than five cases for the

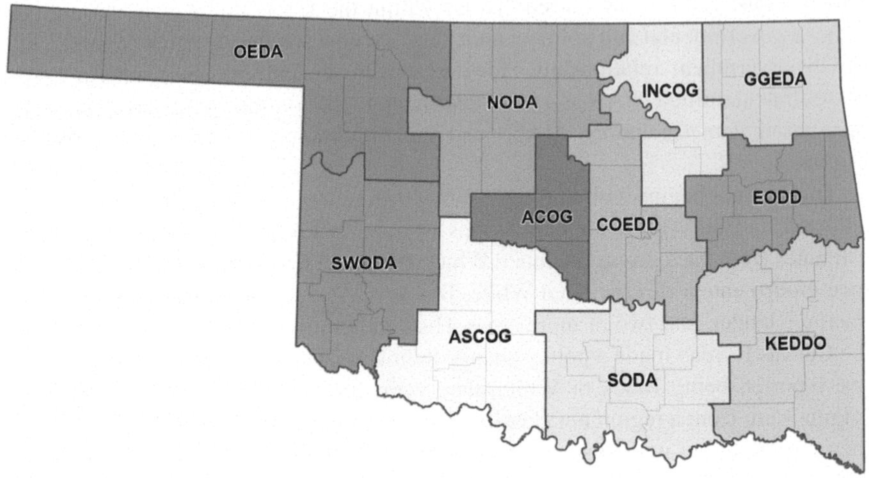

Fig. 1 Substate planning districts (SSPDs) in Oklahoma 2023. Abbreviations: ACOG Association of Central Oklahoma Governments, ASCOG Association of South Central Oklahoma Governments, COEDD Central Oklahoma Economic Development District, EODD Eastern Oklahoma Development District, GGEDA Grand Gateway Economic Development Association, INCOG Indian Nations Council of Governments, KEDDO Kiamichi Economic Development District of Oklahoma, NODA Northern Oklahoma Development Authority, OEDA Oklahoma Economic Development Authority, SODA Southern Oklahoma Development Association, SWODA South Western Oklahoma Developmental Authority

sociodemographic or cancer group. Confidence intervals (CIs) for age-adjusted rates and RRs were determined using the methods outlined by Tiwari et al. (2006). An RR greater than 1.0 signified that the four-race bridged rate surpassed the six-race rate, while an RR less than 1.0 indicated a lower four-race bridged rate compared to the six-race rate. The annual percentage change (APC) was calculated for both four-race bridged and six-race cancer mortality rates to analyze trends from 2010 to 2020 using Joinpoint regression analysis (Statistical Methodology and Applications Branch, 2022). APC was excluded if it relied on fewer than 10 cases for at least one year within the specified time frame. We used an alpha of 0.05 for all analyses.

3 Results

Table 1 presents the differences in deaths and population between the use of four-race and six-race categories. As expected, all single-race categories decreased, accounting for 6.23% of the six-race population classified in the "More than one race" category (Fig. 2).

When reviewing trends over time, no general trend differences were observed; however, differences were noted in APC. Among the White population, the APC for the four-race bridged population estimates was −1.14 (95% CI: −1.6,−0.7), and for

Table 1 Cancer deaths, population estimates, and percent of population by race (Oklahoma 2016–2020)

	Four-race			Six-race		
	Deaths	5-year population estimate	Percent population (%)	Deaths	5-year population estimate	Percent population (%)
Race						
White	34,313	15,288,177	77.47	34,178	14,624,505	74.10
Black or African American	2,594	1,771,464	8.98	2,575	1,535,471	7.78
American Indian or Alaska Native	4,098	2,126,403	10.77	2,769	1,844,010	9.34
Asian*	396	549,214	2.78	325	461,892	2.34
Native Hawaiian or other Pacific Islander*	-	-	-	16	39,876	0.20
Other	-	-	-	650	-	-
Unknown	-	-	-	45	-	-
More than one race	-	-	-	843	1,229,504	6.23
Total	41,401	19,735,258		41,401	19,735,258	

*in Four-race group Asian and Native Hawaiian or Other Pacific Islander are grouped together - represents values that are unavailable

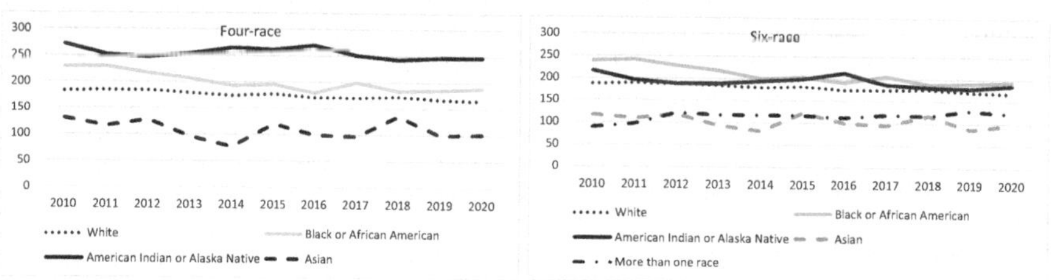

Fig. 2 Trends of cancer mortality rates for four-race and six-race categories by race: Oklahoma 2010–2020

the six-race estimates, −1.18 (95% CI: −1.6,−0.8) (data not shown). There was one Joinpoint for the Black population in 2016. From 2010 to 2016, the four-race bridged APC was −3.64 (95% CI: −7.3, −2.4), and from 2016 to 2020, there was a slight insignificant increase of 0.4 (95% CI: −1.7, 5.3) (data not shown). Using the six-race categories from 2010 to 2014, the APC was −4.7 (95% CI: −9.0, −2.4) for the Black population; from 2014 to 2020, the APC was −1.2 (95% CI: −2.7, 3.3), with the latter period not statistically significant. For the AIAN population, the trend decreased with an APC of −0.54 (95% CI: −1.8, 0.7), and for the six-race categories, the APC was −1.1 (95% CI: −2.3, 0.2); neither trend was statistically significant. However, as shown earlier, the AIAN population using the bridged population estimates had the highest mortality rate of any group. In contrast, the six-race

Table 2 American Indian and Alaska Native six-race vs four-race rate ratio and 95% confidence intervals for cancer mortality using the SEER Site Recode (Oklahoma 2016–2020)

Site	Deaths	AAMRR	95% CI	Site	Deaths	AAMRR	95% CI
Oral cavity and pharynx	54	0.87	(0.52–1.22)	Ovary	98	***0.66***	***(0.45–0.87)***
Esophagus	85	***0.72***	***(0.48–0.96)***	Other female genital system	14	0.67	(0.09–1.25)
Stomach	79	***0.70***	***(0.45–0.95)***	Prostate	175	***0.17***	***(0.15–0.24)***
Small intestine	9	1.00	(0.01–1.99)	Testis	7		
Colon and rectum	449	***0.73***	***(0.63–0.84)***	Other male genital system	<5		
Liver	263	0.84	(0.69–1.00)	Bladder	***70***	***0.72***	***(0.45–0.99)***
Pancreas	234	***0.75***	***(0.60–0.90)***	Kidney and renal pelvis	146	0.84	(0.63–1.05)
Other digestive organs	97	0.81	(0.56–1.06)	Other urinary system	7		
Larynx	33	0.72	(0.34–1.11)	Brain and other nervous system	91	***0.57***	***(0.37–0.77)***
Lung and bronchus	1,061	***0.75***	***(0.68–0.82)***	Thyroid gland	9		
Other respiratory system	11	0.83	(0.07–1.59)	Other endocrine system	7		
Melanomas of the skin	34	***0.45***	***(0.17–0.74)***	Hodgkin lymphoma	10	0.83	(0.03–1.64)
Other skin	28	0.89	(0.39–1.39)	Non-Hodgkin lymphoma	117	***0.70***	***(0.50–0.91)***
Breast	256	***0.42***	***(0.34–0.51)***	Multiple myeloma	86	***0.70***	***(0.46–0.93)***
Cervix uteri	52	0.71	(0.41–1.02)	Leukemias	112	***0.77***	***(0.55–0.99)***
Corpus and uterus, NOS	64	0.76	(0.47–1.06)	Other, ill-defined and unknown	334	***0.77***	***(0.64–0.90)***

AAMRR age-adjusted mortality rate ratio (Six-race vs Four-race)

estimates showed that the Black population had the highest mortality rate. For the Asian population, the trends were decreasing with an APC of −1.31 (95% CI: −5.4, 3.1), and for the six-race categories, the APC was −1.50 (95% CI: −5.0, −2.1) and neither was statistically significant (data not shown). Finally, for the Multiple Race category, there was a significant increase from 2010 to 2012 (APC 15.01, 95% CI: 6.8, 22.5) and a slight increase from 2012 to 2020, as shown by an APC of 0.64 (95% CI: −1.1, 1.6) (data not shown).

When reviewing specific cancers among AIAN populations, only cancer of the small intestine showed no difference between the four-race bridged rates and the six-race denominators (Table 2). A few cancers, particularly those with small numbers, including oral cavity and pharynx ($n = 54$), liver ($n = 263$), other digestive organs ($n = 97$), larynx ($n = 33$), other respiratory systems ($n = 11$), other female genital systems ($n = 14$), bladder ($n = 70$), and kidney and renal pelvis ($n = 146$) show lower RRs, but they were not statistically significant. Additionally, the number of cases for several cancers was too small to permit calculation of mortality rates, including testis ($n = 7$), other male genital systems ($n < 5$), other urinary system ($n = 7$), thyroid gland ($n = 9$), and other endocrine system ($n = 7$). The remaining cancers (esophagus, stomach, colorectal, pancreas, lung and bronchus, melanomas of the skin, breast, ovary, prostate, brain and other nervous system, non-Hodgkin lymphoma, multiple myeloma, leukemias and other, ill-defined and unknown) showed a statistically significant lower RR between the four-race bridged and the six-race categories for the AIAN population.

When examining the geographic distribution around the state, Black and Asian populations showed no significant difference (Table 3). Among White populations, only one substate planning district (GGEDA) showed a small significantly increased rate ratio (1.06; 95% CI: 1.01, 1.11) with the updated six-race denominator data. However, among AIAN populations, 9 of the 11 districts showed significantly lower rates using the updated six-race data. All the districts showed a RR of less than one, ranging from 0.60 to 0.86.

4 Discussion

While overall cancer rate changes were higher for White and Black populations and lower for Asians, these differences were not statistically significant. For the AIAN population, the RR significantly lower when the six-race categories were used. Trends over time showed variations in APC for specific racial groups, with significant lower cancer rates observed among the AIAN population. Specific cancers exhibited a general pattern of lower RR for AIAN populations.

Race is a sociopolitical concept (Braveman & Dominguez, 2021; Gravlee, 2009). Race is not a biological fact, but rather it is a human-invented classification system (Bamshad et al., 2004; Braveman & Dominguez, 2021; Haeny & Polimanti, 2022; Maglo et al., 2016; Mersha & Abebe, 2015). No gene or cluster of genes is common to all individuals of a particular race (Bamshad et al., 2004; Maglo et al., 2016). The concept of race exhibits significant intersociety, within-society, and historical variability (Bamshad et al., 2004). In different societies, and even within societies, racial classifications for individuals can become fluid. For example, a person may be seen by the broader society as White but be politically affiliated as AIAN. Moreover, a person's race can depend on the context. A person may primarily identify as White in society but also be eligible for I/T/Us health care, where they identify as AIAN. This fluidity of racial identity demonstrates even more profoundly that race is a social concept. Moreover, the social, political, and economic meanings of belonging to racial groups have been changing. For instance, the concept of hypodescent in the US, where a biracial person is categorized fully or primarily in terms

Table 3 Six-race vs four-race rate ratio and 95% confidence intervals for major race groups by substate planning districts (Oklahoma 2016–2020)

	White		Black		American Indian or Alaska Native		Asian	
	AAMRR	95% CI	AAMRR	95% CI	AAMRR	95% CI	AAMRR	95% CI
ACOG	0.84	(0.82–0.87)	1.21	(1.12–1.32)	***0.61***	***(0.52–0.69)***	0.97	(0.78–1.16)
ASCOG	1.02	(0.96–1.07)	1.01	(0.81–1.21)	***0.79***	***(0.64–0.93)***	0.91	(0.46–1.37)
COEDD	1.03	(0.98–1.09)	1.10	(0.77–1.43)	0.86	(0.72–1.00)	0.93	(0.25–1.61)
EODD	1.05	(1.00–1.11)	1.09	(0.88–1.30)	***0.82***	***(0.73–0.90)***	0.84	(0.19–1.48)
GGEDA	***1.06***	***(1.01–1.11)***	1.22	(0.76–1.68)	***0.76***	***(0.66–0.85)***	0.69	(0.00–1.37)
INCOG	1.02	(0.98–1.05)	1.00	(0.89–1.11)	***0.69***	***(0.60–0.78)***	0.93	(0.61–1.25)
KEDDO	1.05	(0.98–1.11)	1.09	(0.76–1.41)	***0.74***	***(0.61–0.86)***		
NODA	1.01	(0.94–1.07)	0.94	(0.49–1.39)	***0.71***	***(0.47–0.94)***		
OEDA	0.99	(0.89–1.10)	2.11	(0.52–3.70)	0.60	(0.00–1.20)		
SODA	1.03	(0.97–1.09)	1.03	(0.73–1.43)	***0.84***	***(0.71–0.98)***	0.72	(0.04–1.40)
SWODA	1.00	(0.91–1.08)	1.11	(0.65–1.56)	***0.56***	***(0.31–0.81)***		

AAMRR age-adjusted mortality rate ratio (Six-race vs Four-race)

of the lower status social group, clearly demonstrates that categorization (e.g., as White, as American Indian) is a sociopolitical concept (Banks & Eberhardt, 1998; Ho et al., 2017). However, recognizing race as a social construct does not make race less "real." Like marriages, which are also social constructions, race has profound legal, cultural, and interpersonal implications. In short, race is a sociopolitical concept because it is a human-invented system used to define and stigmatize physical differences between people. It is not a biological reality, but it has real societal consequences.

In 1990, 80% of the US population reported their race and ethnicity as non-Hispanic White on the census, compared to just 58% in 2020 (United States Census Bureau, 2024a). In fact, over the last decade, the growth in the US population has been among non-White populations (United States Census Bureau, 2024a). In 2020, the percentage of the population that reported multiple races was very high in Oklahoma, with 12.8% of the population reporting two or more races (United States Census Bureau, 2024a). (Overall, the US Census shows increased diversity in the population over the last decades (United States Census Bureau, 2021).

Oklahoma has a unique history and population, particularly for the AIAN population. What is now Oklahoma was previously considered Indian Territory where many Tribal Nations were forcibly relocated from their homelands east of the Mississippi River beginning with the 1830 Indian Removal Act. The General Allotment Act of 1887, also known as The Dawes Act, specifically targeted the citizens of the five largest tribes and created the Dawes Commission to assimilate the AIAN population by dividing communally held Tribal lands into individual allotments, thus weakening the Tribal government by disrupting social structures. The Dawes Rolls, also known as the Final Rolls, created a Tribal roll and a Freedman roll. When the rolls closed in 1907, AIAN populations and some Freedmen were allotted land, with the remaining land being taken by the federal government and settled mostly by persons of European ancestry. Additionally, Oklahoma had Historically Black Towns settled after the Civil War. Thus, in Oklahoma, there was a checkerboard pattern of "racial" groups, as opposed to the more concentrated populations found in the northern plains (albeit with smaller numbers), where virtually the entire reservation population is Native. This has led to Oklahoma being one of the most multi-race, multi-Nation populations in the US. In Oklahoma, 47.3% of those who report multiple races reported at least one as AIAN (United States Census Bureau, 2024b).

These data are publicly available for overlapping years, thus allowing differences using these two denominators to be compared. Oklahoma is unique because the state has regularly and routinely published updated information on I/T/U linked cancer incidence and mortality data. Historically, there were important publications using IHS-linked data. In 2008, a group of articles used I/T/U-linked data to show cancer incidence disparities in the US (Becker et al., 2008; Bliss et al., 2008; Cobb et al., 2008; Espey et al., 2008; Henderson et al., 2008; Jim et al., 2008; Kaur & Hampton, 2008; Lemrow et al., 2008; Perdue et al., 2008; Reichman et al., 2008; Steele et al., 2008; Weir et al., 2008; Wiggins et al., 2008a, b; Wilson et al., 2008; Wingo et al., 2008). In 2014, a group of articles with IHS-linked mortality data was completed (Espey et al., 2014a, b; Ford et al., 2014; Groom et al., 2014; Herne et al., 2014; Hoffman et al., 2014; Howard et al., 2014; Ishikawa et al., 2014; Jim et al., 2014; Kaufman et al., 2014; Kunitz et al., 2014; Landen et al., 2014; Li et al., 2014; Murphy et al., 2014; Perdue et al., 2014; Reilley et al., 2014; Rhoades & Rhoades, 2014; Roubideaux & Karol, 2014; Schieb et al., 2014; Singh et al., 2014; Suryaprasad et al., 2014; Veazie et al., 2014; Warne & Frizzell, 2014; Watson et al., 2014; White et al., 2014a). These works would benefit from comprehensive updating but that may not be possible given the issues discussed here.

5 Conclusions

Analyzing data is crucial for making informed decisions. As our societies evolve, it is essential to update data to reflect these changes, but we must proceed with caution. Researchers have a responsibility to thoroughly understand and clearly explain changes in population estimates and their implications. This is not just for fellow researchers—it is essential for policymakers and society as a whole so that attention and resources can be accurately focused.

It is important to continue informing researchers, policy makers, and the general population that race is a social construct and classifying AIAN people as a race is a historical error that deserves correction. Moreover, with each proposed change to population estimates, we may further misclassify population groups, potentially influencing population-level estimates of risk and mortality. When examining AIAN rates, researchers must be meticulous in understanding and explaining the sources for both the numerator and the denominator.

Disseminating these results effectively is key to addressing the true burden of cancer among AIAN populations. Using Oklahoma as an example, a significant difference emerged due to a change in policy. While this change is necessary for a better understanding of the US's diverse populations, we must fully grasp its potential negative impacts on reporting.

Acknowledgments We extend our sincere gratitude to Oklahoma Vital Records for their years of dedication to maintaining accurate, transparent, and accessible public health data. Their commitment to data integrity has been invaluable in advancing research and informing public health policies. The availability of high-quality mortality data through Oklahoma Statistics on Health Available for Everyone (OK2SHARE) has enabled the analysis and understanding of critical health trends, particularly among historically underrepresented populations.

We also acknowledge the efforts of the individuals and teams who meticulously collect, manage, and maintain these vital records. Their work ensures that researchers, policymakers, and the public have access to reliable data to inform decision-making and improve health outcomes.

Finally, we recognize the many individuals and families whose health experiences are reflected in these records. Their data contributes to a greater understanding of public health challenges and helps drive meaningful change.

This research is supported by the National Institute of General Medical Sciences, Grant/Award Number: U5GM104938 awarded to the University of Oklahoma Health Campus, U19 MDO20537 awarded to the University of Oklahoma Stephenson Cancer Center, and the National Cancer

Institute Cancer Center Support Grant P30CA225520 awarded to the University of Oklahoma Stephenson Cancer Center and used the Stephenson Cancer Center Biostatistics and Research Design Shared Resource. The content is solely the authors' responsibility and does not necessarily represent the official views of the The University of Oklahoma Health Campus, National Institutes of Health, or the Stephenson Cancer Center.

Declarations of Interest None.

Consent to Participate This was a secondary data analysis of de-identified online surveillance data. Therefore, the The University of Oklahoma Health Campus IRB deemed informed consent unnecessary.

Availability of Data and Materials (Data Transparency) Data are available from the **Ok**lahoma **S**tatistics on **H**ealth **A**vailable fo**r** **E**veryone (OK2SHARE) and are publicly accessible.

References

Allen, J. P., & Turner, E. (2001). Bridging 1990 and 2000 census race data: Fractional assignment of multiracial populations. *Population Research and Policy Review, 20*(6), 513–533. https://doi.org/10.1023/A:1015666321798

Amodio, E., Zarcone, M., Casuccio, A., & Vitale, F. (2021). Trends in epidemiology: The role of denominator fluctuation in population based estimates. *AIMS Public Health, 8*(3), 500–506. https://doi.org/10.3934/publichealth.2021040

Bamshad, M., Wooding, S., Salisbury, B. A., & Stephens, J. C. (2004). Deconstructing the relationship between genetics and race. *Nature Reviews Genetics, 5*(8), 598–609. https://doi.org/10.1038/nrg1401

Banks, R. R., & Eberhardt, J. L. (1998). Social psychological processes and the legal bases of racial categorization. In J. Eberhardt & S. Fisk (Eds.), *Confronting racism: The problem and the response* (pp. 54–75).

Becker, T. M., Espey, D. K., Lawson, H. W., Saraiya, M., Jim, M. A., & Waxman, A. G. (2008). Regional differences in cervical cancer incidence among American Indians and Alaska Natives, 1999-2004. *Cancer, 113*(5 Suppl), 1234–1243. https://doi.org/10.1002/cncr.23736

Bliss, A., Cobb, N., Solomon, T., Cravatt, K., Jim, M. A., Marshall, L., & Campbell, J. (2008). Lung cancer incidence among American Indians and Alaska Natives in the United States, 1999-2004. *Cancer, 113*(5 Suppl), 1168–1178. https://doi.org/10.1002/cncr.23738

Braveman, P., & Dominguez, T. P. (2021). Abandon "Race." Focus on racism. *Frontiers in Public Health, 9*, 689462. ARTN 689462. https://doi.org/10.3389/fpubh.2021.689462

Cobb, N., Wingo, P. A., & Edwards, B. K. (2008). Introduction to the supplement on cancer in the American Indian and Alaska Native populations in the United States. *Cancer, 113*(5 Suppl), 1113–1116. https://doi.org/10.1002/cncr.23729

Espey, D. K., Wiggins, C. L., Jim, M. A., Miller, B. A., Johnson, C. J., & Becker, T. M. (2008). Methods for improving cancer surveillance data in American Indian and Alaska Native populations. *Cancer, 113*(5 Suppl), 1120–1130. https://doi.org/10.1002/cncr.23724

Espey, D. K., Jim, M. A., Cobb, N., Bartholomew, M., Becker, T., Haverkamp, D., & Plescia, M. (2014a). Leading causes of death and all-cause mortality in American Indians and Alaska Natives. *American Journal of Public Health, 104 Suppl 3*(Suppl 3), S303–S311. https://doi.org/10.2105/AJPH.2013.301798

Espey, D. K., Jim, M. A., Richards, T. B., Begay, C., Haverkamp, D., & Roberts, D. (2014b). Methods for improving the quality and completeness of mortality data for American Indians and Alaska Natives. *American Journal of Public Health, 104 Suppl 3*(Suppl 3), S286–S294. https://doi.org/10.2105/AJPH.2013.301716

Ford, J. D., Willox, A. C., Chatwood, S., Furgal, C., Harper, S., Mauro, I., & Pearce, T. (2014). Adapting to the effects of climate change on Inuit health [Research Support, Non-U.S. Gov't Review]. *American Journal of Public Health, 104 Suppl3*(Suppl 3), e9–17. https://doi.org/10.2105/AJPH.2013.301724

Frey, W. H. (2021). *New 2020 census results show increased diversity countering decade-long declines in America's white and youth populations*. https://policycommons.net/artifacts/4145163/new-2020-census-results-show-increased-diversity-countering-decade-long-declines-in-americas-white-and-youth-populations/

Gravlee, C. C. (2009). How race becomes biology: Embodiment of social inequality. *American Journal of Physical Anthropology, 139*(1), 47–57. https://doi.org/10.1002/ajpa.20983

Groom, A. V., Hennessy, T. W., Singleton, R. J., Butler, J. C., Holve, S., & Cheek, J. E. (2014). Pneumonia and influenza mortality among American Indian and Alaska Native people, 1990-2009 [Comparative Study]. *American Journal of Public Health, 104 Suppl 3*(Suppl 3), S460–S469. https://doi.org/10.2105/AJPH.2013.301740

Haeny, A. M., & Polimanti, R. (2022). From evolutionary history to the concepts of race and ancestry: Shifting our perspective in clinical research. *Biological Psychiatry, 91*(12), e51–e52. https://doi.org/10.1016/j.biopsych.2022.02.953

Haozous, E. A., Strickland, C. J., Palacios, J. F., & Solomon, T. G. (2014). Blood politics, ethnic identity, and racial misclassification among American Indians and Alaska Natives. *Journal of Environmental and Public Health, 2014*, 321604. https://doi.org/10.1155/2014/321604

Haring, R. C., Jim, M. A., Erwin, D., Kaur, J., Henry, W. A. E., Haring, M. L., & Seneca, D. S. (2018). Mortality disparities: A comparison with the Haudenosaunee in New York State. *Cancer Health Disparities, 2*. https://doi.org/10.9777/chd.2018.10009

Henderson, J. A., Espey, D. K., Jim, M. A., German, R. R., Shaw, K. M., & Hoffman, R. M. (2008). Prostate cancer incidence among American Indian and Alaska Native men, US, 1999-2004. *Cancer, 113*(5 Suppl), 1203–1212. https://doi.org/10.1002/cncr.23739

Herne, M. A., Bartholomew, M. L., & Weahkee, R. L. (2014). Suicide mortality among American Indians and Alaska Natives, 1999-2009. *American Journal of Public Health, 104 Suppl 3*(Suppl 3), S336–S342. https://doi.org/10.2105/AJPH.2014.301929

Ho, A. K., Kteily, N. S., & Chen, J. M. (2017). "You're One of Us": Black Americans' use of Hypodescent and its association with egalitarianism. *Journal of Personality and Social Psychology, 113*(5), 753–768. https://doi.org/10.1037/pspi0000107

Hoffman, R. M., Li, J., Henderson, J. A., Ajani, U. A., & Wiggins, C. (2014). Prostate cancer deaths and incident cases among American Indian/Alaska Native men, 1999-2009 [Comparative Study Research Support N.I.H., Extramural]. *American Journal of Public Health, 104 Suppl 3*(Suppl 3), S439–S445. https://doi.org/10.2105/AJPH.2013.301690

Howard, B. V., Metzger, J. S., Koller, K. R., Jolly, S. E., Asay, E. D., Wang, H., Wolfe, A. W., Hopkins, S. E., Kaufmann, C., Raymer, T. W., Trimble, B., Provost, E. M., Ebbesson, S. O., Austin, M. A., Howard, W. J., Umans, J. G., & Boyer, B. B. (2014). All-cause, cardiovascular, and cancer mortality in western Alaska Native people: Western Alaska Tribal Collaborative for Health (WATCH). *American Journal of Public Health, 104*(7), 1334–1340. https://doi.org/10.2105/AJPH.2013.301614

Ingram, D. D., Parker, J. D., Schenker, N., Weed, J. A., Hamilton, B. E., Arias, E., & Madans, J. H. (2003). US census 2000 population with bridged race categories.

Ishikawa, T., Oudie, E., Desapriya, E., Turcotte, K., & Pike, I. (2014). A systematic review of community interventions to improve Aboriginal child passenger safety [Comparative Study Research Support, N.I.H., Extramural]. *American Journal of Public Health, 104 Suppl 3*(Suppl 3), e1–e8. https://doi.org/10.2105/AJPH.2013.301683

Jim, M. A., Perdue, D. G., Richardson, L. C., Espey, D. K., Redd, J. T., Martin, H. J., Kwong, S. L., Kelly, J. J., Henderson, J. A., & Ahmed, F. (2008). Primary liver cancer incidence among American Indians and Alaska Natives, US, 1999-2004. *Cancer, 113*(5 Suppl), 1244–1255. https://doi.org/10.1002/cncr.23728

Jim, M. A., Arias, E., Seneca, D. S., Hoopes, M. J., Jim, C. C., Johnson, N. J., & Wiggins, C. L. (2014). Racial misclassification of American Indians and Alaska Natives by Indian Health

Service Contract Health Service Delivery Area. *American Journal of Public Health, 104 Suppl 3*(Suppl 3), S295–S302. https://doi.org/10.2105/AJPH.2014.301933

Kaufman, C. E., Whitesell, N. R., Keane, E. M., Desserich, J. A., Giago, C., Sam, A., & Mitchell, C. M. (2014). Effectiveness of Circle of Life, an HIV-preventive intervention for American Indian middle school youths: A group randomized trial in a Northern Plains tribe. *American Journal of Public Health, 104*(6), e106–e112. https://doi.org/10.2105/AJPH.2013.301822

Kaur, J. S., & Hampton, J. W. (2008). Cancer in American Indian and Alaska Native populations continues to threaten an aging population: The need for tribal, state, and federal action. *Cancer, 113*(5 Suppl), 1117–1119. https://doi.org/10.1002/cncr.23730

Kills First, C. C., Sutton, T. L., Shannon, J., Brody, J. R., & Sheppard, B. C. (2022). Disparities in pancreatic cancer care and research in Native Americans: Righting a history of wrongs [Research Support, N.I.H., Extramural Research Support, Non-U.S. Gov't]. *Cancer, 128*(8), 1560–1567. https://doi.org/10.1002/cncr.34118

Kratzer, T. B., Jemal, A., Miller, K. D., Nash, S., Wiggins, C., Redwood, D., Smith, R., & Siegel, R. L. (2022). Cancer statistics for American Indian and Alaska Native individuals, 2022: Including increasing disparities in early onset colorectal cancer [Review]. *CA: a Cancer Journal for Clinicians*. https://doi.org/10.3322/caac.21757

Kunitz, S. J., Veazie, M., & Henderson, J. A. (2014). Historical trends and regional differences in all-cause and amenable mortality among American Indians and Alaska Natives since 1950. *American Journal of Public Health, 104 Suppl 3*(Suppl 3), S268–S277. https://doi.org/10.2105/AJPH.2013.301684

Landen, M., Roeber, J., Naimi, T., Nielsen, L., & Sewell, M. (2014). Alcohol-attributable mortality among American Indians and Alaska Natives in the United States, 1999-2009. *American Journal of Public Health, 104 Suppl 3*(Suppl 3), S343–S349. https://doi.org/10.2105/AJPH.2013.301648

Layne, T. M., Ferrucci, L. M., Jones, B. A., Smith, T., Gonsalves, L., & Cartmel, B. (2019). Concordance of cancer registry and self-reported race, ethnicity, and cancer type: A report from the American Cancer Society's studies of cancer survivors. *Cancer Causes & Control, 30*(1), 21–29. https://doi.org/10.1007/s10552-018-1091-3

Lemrow, S. M., Perdue, D. G., Stewart, S. L., Richardson, L. C., Jim, M. A., French, H. T., Swan, J., Edwards, B. K., Wiggins, C., Dickie, L., & Espey, D. K. (2008). Gallbladder cancer incidence among American Indians and Alaska Natives, US, 1999-2004. *Cancer, 113*(5 Suppl), 1266–1273. https://doi.org/10.1002/cncr.23737

Li, J., Weir, H. K., Jim, M. A., King, S. M., Wilson, R., & Master, V. A. (2014). Kidney cancer incidence and mortality among American Indians and Alaska Natives in the United States, 1990-2009 [Comparative Study]. *American Journal of Public Health, 104 Suppl 3*(Suppl 3), S396–S403. https://doi.org/10.2105/AJPH.2013.301616

Llaneza, A. J., Holt, A., Seward, J., Piatt, J., & Campbell, J. E. (2024). Assessment of racial misclassification among American Indian and Alaska Native identity in cancer surveillance data in the United States and considerations for oral health: A systematic review. *Health Equity, 8*(1), 376–390. https://doi.org/10.1089/heq.2023.0252

Maglo, K. N., Mersha, T. B., & Martin, L. J. (2016). Population genomics and the statistical values of race: An interdisciplinary perspective on the biological classification of human populations and implications for clinical genetic epidemiological research. *Frontiers in Genetics, 7*, 22. https://doi.org/10.3389/fgene.2016.00022

Melkonian, S. C., Jim, M. A., Pete, D., Poel, A., Dominguez, A. E., Echo-Hawk, A., Zhang, S., Wilson, R. J., Haverkamp, D., Petras, L., & Pohlenz, A. (2022). Cancer disparities among non-Hispanic urban American Indian and Alaska Native populations in the United States, 1999-2017. *Cancer, 128*(8), 1626–1636. https://doi.org/10.1002/cncr.34122

Mersha, T. B., & Abebe, T. (2015). Self-reported race/ethnicity in the age of genomic research: Its potential impact on understanding health disparities. *Human Genomics, 9*(1), 1. https://doi.org/10.1186/s40246-014-0023-x

Michalek, A. M., Mahoney, M. C., Cummings, K. M., Hanley, J., & Snyder, R. (1989). Mortality patterns among a Native American population in New York State. *New York State Journal of Medicine, 89*(10), 557–561. https://www.ncbi.nlm.nih.gov/pubmed/2608215

Murphy, T., Pokhrel, P., Worthington, A., Billie, H., Sewell, M., & Bill, N. (2014). Unintentional injury mortality among American Indians and Alaska Natives in the United States, 1990-2009. *American Journal of Public Health, 104 Suppl 3*(Suppl 3), S470–S480. https://doi.org/10.2105/AJPH.2013.301854

Parker, J. D., Schenker, N., Ingram, D. D., Weed, J. A., Heck, K. E., & Madans, J. H. (2004). Bridging between two standards for collecting information on race and ethnicity: An application to Census 2000 and vital rates. *Public Health Reports, 119*(2), 192–205. https://doi.org/10.1177/003335490411900213

Perdue, D. G., Perkins, C., Jackson-Thompson, J., Coughlin, S. S., Ahmed, F., Haverkamp, D. S., & Jim, M. A. (2008). Regional differences in colorectal cancer incidence, stage, and subsite among American Indians and Alaska Natives, 1999-2004. *Cancer, 113*(5 Suppl), 1179–1190. https://doi.org/10.1002/cncr.23726

Perdue, D. G., Haverkamp, D., Perkins, C., Daley, C. M., & Provost, E. (2014). Geographic variation in colorectal cancer incidence and mortality, age of onset, and stage at diagnosis among American Indian and Alaska Native people, 1990-2009 [Comparative Study]. *American Journal of Public Health, 104 Suppl 3*(Suppl 3), S404–S414. https://doi.org/10.2105/AJPH.2013.301654

Plescia, M., Henley, S. J., Pate, A., Underwood, J. M., & Rhodes, K. (2014). Lung cancer deaths among American Indians and Alaska Natives, 1990-2009 [Comparative Study]. *American Journal of Public Health, 104 Suppl 3*(Suppl 3), S388–S395. https://doi.org/10.2105/AJPH.2013.301609

Reichman, M. E., Kelly, J. J., Kosary, C. L., Coughlin, S. S., Jim, M. A., & Lanier, A. P. (2008). Incidence of cancers of the oral cavity and pharynx among American Indians and Alaska Natives, 1999-2004. *Cancer, 113*(5 Suppl), 1256–1265. https://doi.org/10.1002/cncr.23735

Reilley, B., Bloss, E., Byrd, K. K., Iralu, J., Neel, L., & Cheek, J. (2014). Death rates from human immunodeficiency virus and tuberculosis among American Indians/Alaska Natives in the United States, 1990-2009 [Comparative Study]. *American Journal of Public Health, 104 Suppl 3*(Suppl 3), S453–S459. https://doi.org/10.2105/AJPH.2013.301746

Rhee, C., & Klompas, M. (2020). Sepsis trends: Increasing incidence and decreasing mortality, or changing denominator? *Journal of Thoracic Disease, 12*(Suppl 1), S89–S100. https://doi.org/10.21037/jtd.2019.12.51

Rhoades, E. R., & Rhoades, D. A. (2014). The public health foundation of health services for American Indians & Alaska Natives [Historical Article]. *American Journal of Public Health, 104 Suppl 3*(Suppl 3), S278–S285. https://doi.org/10.2105/AJPH.2013.301767

Roubideaux, Y., & Karol, S. V. (2014). Perspectives on mortality data from the Indian Health Service [Introductory]. *American Journal of Public Health, 104 Suppl 3*(Suppl 3), S254. https://doi.org/10.2105/AJPH.2014.301987

Schieb, L. J., Ayala, C., Valderrama, A. L., & Veazie, M. A. (2014). Trends and disparities in stroke mortality by region for American Indians and Alaska Natives [Comparative Study]. *American Journal of Public Health, 104 Suppl 3*(Suppl 3), S368–S376. https://doi.org/10.2105/AJPH.2013.301698

Singh, S. D., Ryerson, A. B., Wu, M., & Kaur, J. S. (2014). Ovarian and uterine cancer incidence and mortality in American Indian and Alaska Native women, United States, 1999-2009 [Comparative Study]. *American Journal of Public Health, 104 Suppl 3*(Suppl 3), S423–S431. https://doi.org/10.2105/AJPH.2013.301781

Starr, P., & Pao, C. (2024). The multiracial complication: The 2020 census and the fictitious multiracial boom. *Sociological Science, 11*, 1107–1123. https://doi.org/10.15195/v11.a40

Statistical Methodology and Applications Branch, S. R. P., National Cancer Institute. (2022). *Joinpoint Regression Program, Version 4.9.1.0*. In (Version 4.9.1.0) https://surveillance.cancer.gov/help/joinpoint

Statistics, N. C. f. H. (2003). *United States Census 2000 population with bridged race categories*. National Center for Health Statistics.

Steele, C. B., Cardinez, C. J., Richardson, L. C., Tom-Orme, L., & Shaw, K. M. (2008). Surveillance for health behaviors of American Indians and Alaska Natives-findings from the behavioral risk factor surveillance system, 2000-2006. *Cancer, 113*(5 Suppl), 1131–1141. https://doi.org/10.1002/cncr.23727

Stehr-Green, P., Bettles, J., & Robertson, L. D. (2002). Effect of racial/ethnic misclassification of American Indians and Alaskan Natives on Washington State death certificates, 1989-1997. *American Journal of Public Health, 92*(3), 443–444. https://doi.org/10.2105/ajph.92.3.443

Suryaprasad, A., Byrd, K. K., Redd, J. T., Perdue, D. G., Manos, M. M., & McMahon, B. J. (2014). Mortality caused by chronic liver disease among American Indians and Alaska Natives in the United States, 1999-2009 [Comparative Study Research Support, N.I.H., Extramural]. *American Journal of Public Health, 104 Suppl3*(Suppl 3), S350–S358. https://doi.org/10.2105/AJPH.2013.301645

Tiwari, R. C., Clegg, L. X., & Zou, Z. (2006). Efficient interval estimation for age-adjusted cancer rates. *Statistical Methods in Medical Research, 15*(6), 547–569. https://doi.org/10.1177/0962280206070621

United States Census Bureau. (2017). *American Community survey information guide*. Retrieved from https://www.census.gov/content/dam/Census/programs-surveys/acs/about/ACS_Information_Guide.pdf

United States Census Bureau. (2021). *Improved race and ethnicity measures reveal US* (Population Is Much More Multiracial. United States Census Bureau., Issue. https://www.census.gov/library/stories/2021/08/improve d-race-ethnicity-measures-reveal-united-states-population-much-more-multiracial. html2021

United States Census Bureau. (2024a). *Data and maps*. www.census.gov

United States Census Bureau. (2024b). *U.S. Census Bureau, 2023 American Community Survey*. Retrieved February 20 from https://www.census.gov/

Veazie, M., Ayala, C., Schieb, L., Dai, S., Henderson, J. A., & Cho, P. (2014). Trends and disparities in heart disease mortality among American Indians/Alaska Natives, 1990-2009 [Comparative Study Research Support, N.I.H., Extramural]. *American Journal of Public Health, 104 Suppl 3*(Suppl 3), S359–S367. https://doi.org/10.2105/AJPH.2013.301715

Warne, D., & Frizzell, L. B. (2014). American Indian health policy: Historical trends and contemporary issues [Historical Article]. *American Journal of Public Health, 104 Suppl 3*(Suppl 3), S263–S267. https://doi.org/10.2105/AJPH.2013.301682

Watson, M., Benard, V., Thomas, C., Brayboy, A., Paisano, R., & Becker, T. (2014). Cervical cancer incidence and mortality among American Indian and Alaska Native women, 1999-2009 [Comparative Study]. *American Journal of Public Health, 104 Suppl 3*(Suppl 3), S415–S422. https://doi.org/10.2105/AJPH.2013.301681

Weir, H. K., Jim, M. A., Marrett, L. D., & Fairley, T. (2008). Cancer in American Indian and Alaska native young adults (ages 20-44 years): US, 1999-2004 [Research Support, U.S. Gov't, P.H.S.]. *Cancer, 113*(5 Suppl), 1153–1167. https://doi.org/10.1002/cncr.23731

White, A., Richardson, L. C., Li, C., Ekwueme, D. U., & Kaur, J. S. (2014a). Breast cancer mortality among American Indian and Alaska Native women, 1990-2009 [Comparative Study]. *American Journal of Public Health, 104 Suppl 3*(Suppl 3), S432–S438. https://doi.org/10.2105/AJPH.2013.301720

White, M. C., Espey, D. K., Swan, J., Wiggins, C. L., Eheman, C., & Kaur, J. S. (2014b). Disparities in cancer mortality and incidence among American Indians and Alaska Natives in the United States [Comparative Study Research Support N.I.H., Extramural]. *American Journal of Public Health, 104 Suppl 3*(Suppl 3), S377–S387. https://doi.org/10.2105/AJPH.2013.301673

Wiggins, C. L., Espey, D. K., Wingo, P. A., Kaur, J. S., Wilson, R. T., Swan, J., Miller, B. A., Jim, M. A., Kelly, J. J., & Lanier, A. P. (2008a). Cancer among American Indians and Alaska Natives in the United States, 1999-2004. *Cancer, 113*(5 Suppl), 1142–1152. https://doi.org/10.1002/cncr.23734

Wiggins, C. L., Perdue, D. G., Henderson, J. A., Bruce, M. G., Lanier, A. P., Kelley, J. J., Seals, B. F., & Espey, D. K. (2008b). Gastric cancer among American Indians and Alaska Natives in the United States, 1999-2004. *Cancer, 113*(5 Suppl), 1225–1233. https://doi.org/10.1002/cncr.23732

Wilson, R. T., Richardson, L. C., Kelly, J. J., Kaur, J., Jim, M. A., & Lanier, A. P. (2008). Cancers of the urinary tract among American Indians and Alaska Natives in the United States, 1999-2004. *Cancer, 113*(5 Suppl), 1213–1224. https://doi.org/10.1002/cncr.23733

Wingo, P. A., King, J., Swan, J., Coughlin, S. S., Kaur, J. S., Erb-Alvarez, J. A., Jackson-Thompson, J., & Arambula Solomon, T. G. (2008). Breast cancer incidence among American Indian and Alaska Native women: US, 1999-2004. *Cancer, 113*(5 Suppl), 1191–1202. https://doi.org/10.1002/cncr.23725

Yankaskas, B. C., Knight, K. L., Fleg, A., & Rao, C. (2009). Misclassification of American Indian race in state cancer data among non-federally recognized Indians in North Carolina [Comparative Study Research Support, N.I.H., Extramural Research Support, U.S. Gov't, P.H.S.]. *Journal of Registry Management, 36*(1), 7–11. https://www.ncbi.nlm.nih.gov/pubmed/19670692

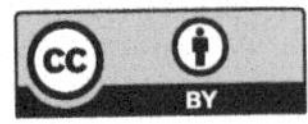

Adapting Cancer Health Literacy Materials for Indigenous Populations: A Literature Review and Exemplar Quality Improvement Project

Wehonna Toth, Michelle Huyser, Regina Mowry, Emma Villeneuve, Caitlin Persico, Whitney Ann E. Henry, Ja:no's-Janine Bowen, Brenda White-Battleson, Kris Rhodes, Will Maybee, and Rodney C. Haring

Abstract Quality improvement (QI) focused on the review and refinement of outreach materials is important for enhancing Indigenous health care. Here, a health literacy QI project is described involving the incorporation of Indigenous knowledge into cancer prevention outreach materials. Indigenous peoples face some of

W. Toth
Department of Nursing, University of Colorado, Clinical Services, UCHealth, Colorado Springs, CO, USA

M. Huyser
University of Missouri, Department of Surgery, Surgical Oncology Division, Columbia, MO, USA

R. Mowry
Department of Health Sciences, Daemen University, Community Health Programs, Roswell Park Comprehensive Cancer Center, Buffalo, NY, USA

E. Villeneuve
Faculty of Education, McMaster University, Hamilton, ON, Canada

C. Persico
School of Nursing, University at Buffalo, Buffalo, NY, USA

W. A. E. Henry · W. Maybee · R. C. Haring (✉)
Department of Indigenous Cancer Health, Roswell Park Comprehensive Cancer Center, Buffalo, NY, USA
e-mail: Rodney.Haring@RoswellPark.org

J.-J. Bowen
Doctor of Educational Leadership Program, D'Youville University, Buffalo, NY, USA

B. White-Battleson
Department of Information Science, University at Buffalo, Buffalo, NY, USA

K. Rhodes
Office of American Indian Health and Tribal Relations, Minnesota Department of Health, St Paul, MN, USA

R. C. Haring (ed.), *Indigenous Genetics, Biobanking, Chemistry, and Cancer Research*, Cancer Health Disparities, https://doi.org/10.1007/978-3-032-17296-9_7

the greatest health disparities globally, including increased rates of cancer diagnoses at later stages and higher mortality rates than the general population. Student interns from a US National Cancer Institute (NCI)-designated cancer center and Canadian University shared responsibility in working with Indigenous first-language speakers over multiple summers to improve messaging. For Indigenous populations, usable, visually appealing, and culturally sensitive information are key to communicating important messages. Outreach materials then underwent elder review, creating new language definitions for use in English-to-Indigenous language adaptations. Next, the cancer center's creative service team produced revised materials incorporating recommendations. Finally, the materials were presented back to Black, Indigenous, People of Color (BIPOC) urban community groups and allies. Reviewers noted the importance of community-friendly language and incorporation of Indigenous language. Increased use of Indigenous-based cancer statistics and delivery of Indigenous-adapted materials back to health systems, urban centers, and community-based organizations were recommended. These experiences offer an exemplar to strengthen tribal programming.

Keywords Quality improvement · Data sharing · Cancer prevention · Health literacy · Indigenous · Language · Health disparities · Outreach

1 Quality Improvement as a Tool for Achieving Improvements in Population Health

Both research and quality improvement projects are important for achieving improvements in population health. Research is a scientific process that is used to generate evidence-based knowledge beneficial to research participants and the larger scientific community (Beyea & Nicoll, 1998). Research projects usually are hypotheses driven, are guided by a study design, follow rigorous methods, and have an end goal of the generation of new scientific knowledge (Beyea & Nicoll, 1998). Due to potential risks to participants, research involving human subjects must be reviewed and approved by an Institutional Review Board (IRB), which functions as an ethics committee to ensure human participation in such research is safe and ethical (Grady, 2015), both domestically and internationally. Researchers must be qualified and approved by the IRB (Mertens, 1998 in Reinhardt & Ray, 2003), and the IRB review and approval process can take up to a month or more. Quality improvement (QI) initiatives are carried out to evaluate and improve on existing services or programming (Reinhardt & Ray, 2003), and QI projects are viable way to address many needs in health care settings safely and effectively (Beyea & Nicoll, 1998). This project describes a health literacy QI project involving the incorporation of Indigenous knowledge into cancer prevention outreach materials, through extensive collaborations with Indigenous first-language speakers, elders, and community groups.

2 Health Literacy as a Foundation for Wellness in Indigenous Populations

Health literacy refers to the capacity of a person to understand health issues in relation to reliable literature, writings, and other readable documents. In the context of this chapter, American Indian, Alaska Native, Native American, First Nations, and Metis are used interchangeably as Indigenous and are reflective of the original peoples of North America. Tribes and Native Nations are also interchangeable definitions representing sovereign Indigenous Nations. Health literacy QI projects focused on cancer prevention and screening were identified as high priority by the Department of Indigenous Cancer Health at Roswell Park Comprehensive Cancer Center in Buffalo, New York. Cancer is an important health issue among Indigenous peoples, along with cardiovascular disease, and health disparities are prevalent in Indigenous populations (Brega et al., 2013). Globally, Indigenous peoples face some of the greatest health disparities, including increased rates of cancer diagnoses at later stages and higher mortality rates than the general population. In the Great Lakes region, cancer is the second-leading cause of death for the Haudenosaunee (Iroquois) (Haring et al., 2018). Cancer and health disparities among Indigenous peoples are multifaceted, but poor understanding of health information can be a contributing factor.

Several useful definitions and foundational studies on health literacy exist. Brega et al. (2013) define health literacy as "the capacity to obtain, process, and understand basic health information and services needed to make appropriate health decisions." Lambert et al. (2014) explains health literacy as the "ability to access, understand, evaluate and communicate information as a way to promote, maintain and improve health in a variety of settings across the life-course" (Rootman & Gordon-El-Bihbety, 2008, as cited in Lambert et al., 2014, p. 2). More broadly, health literacy impacts communities differently based on their understanding of health care, cultural beliefs about health care, and language related to health (Keleher & Hagger, 2007). As described by the Canadian Expert Panel on Health, 48% of Indigenous adults have limited health literacy skills, which significantly limits disease prevention, diagnosis, treatment, and survival (Kutner et al., 2006). Lambert et al. (2014) explained that those with a high level of health literacy tend to use preventative services and seek and comply with treatments, and thus, show improved management of chronic conditions.

3 Findings from the Literature Review

Breast cancer is one area where health literacy improvements could be particularly beneficial. In the Southwest United States, Indigenous women have a significantly lower age-adjusted breast cancer incidence rate than non-Hispanic White women (Espey et al., 2007); although these rates represent a positive health trend for

Indigenous women, studies have shown that Indigenous women are frequently diagnosed at later stages of cancer and have the lowest breast cancer survival rates (as cited in Yost et al., 2017). Also, as discussed by Yost et al. (2017) and based on previous studies, noncompliance in mammography screening, barriers in cancer communication, and emotional distress can potentially result in a late diagnosis, leading to worse outcomes. For Indigenous women to be successful at obtaining screening services like breast mammography, they need to be aware and understand the benefits of screening, and their perceived barriers to obtaining them must be addressed by health care providers/systems (Roh et al., 2018). Furthermore, to improve modifiable cancer outcomes within Indigenous communities, they need to be able to navigate, communicate, and participate in their complex cancer care, which is lacking in many of these communities due to health literacy deficiencies (Thewes et al., 2018).

While health literacy is important to change individual behavior, the broader community in which one resides can impact health care improvement efforts and community literacy (Jones et al., 2020). A Canadian literacy systematic review identified that many Indigenous peoples make cancer treatment decisions based on significant others and extended family, not just as an individual (Thewes et al., 2018). Effective health communications grounded in context and held beliefs have been shown to encourage positive health behaviors and adherence to medical therapies and reduce anxiety about health treatments (Cassady, 2008, as cited in Boyd et al., 2021). Furthermore, intergenerational knowledge sharing among Indigenous families, both genetic and kinship, have been shown to influence health-related behaviors (Smith et al., 2020). These examples highlight the importance of community considerations when formulating health literacy interventions. Another example that underscores the importance of these findings involves the Diné (Navajo), a southwestern Indigenous community, who work better together through families and kinship rather than as individuals. Group values and relationships have created strong cultural ties among the community for many generations (Yost et al., 2017). The most primal and prominent of the Diné culture is the language. Although mostly spoken, the written language has evolved over time. Fundamental to understanding health care remains the ability to understand health-related language (Thewes et al., 2018). Health interventions can fail due to participant difficulty understanding medical words or limited use of visual aids (Lakhan et al., 2017).

In research conducted by Hoffman-Goetz and Friedman (2007), the participating Indigenous (from Canada) women expressed that it was essential for everyone, Indigenous or not, to access, read, and understand health-related information to prevent illness and treat disease symptoms. Many Indigenous languages lack a word for cancer or describe it as a single disease with a single morbid outcome, despite various types of cancer and outcomes (Thewes et al., 2018). To increase health literacy within the Diné, translators created definitions for clinical words such as the term *cancer*. It is unlikely that literal translations of words and meanings will occur in many Indigenous languages. For example, the term *cancer* in Diné, *lhóód doo nádzihii*, directly translates to "the sore that does not heal" (Csordas, 1989, as cited in Yost et al., 2017). However, such translations may lead to misunderstanding among the community. For instance, a "sore that does not heal" may suggest to some that cancer is incurable and therefore seeking medical treatment would be useless. Similar efforts utilizing a "two-eyed seeing approach" has been used to decolonize health information by stressing the importance of both Indigenous cultural and Western concepts being harmonious, even if no direct translation exists (Webkamigad et al., 2020). It is important that when one does translate terms from one language to another, that the term can translate forward and backward. It is also important that translations do not cause a misconception of a term but rather provide a clear and accurate definition.

Other studies have examined the role of Indigenous language barriers in health literacy and behavior among Indigenous populations. In most of these, Indigenous language usage was measured in concert with other components of Indigenous tradition and culture. Studies have found that many Indigenous communities believe cancer is a product of an unhealthy lifestyle or deviating from traditional beliefs (Thewes et al., 2018). The degree to which Indigenous peoples identify with their traditional cultural beliefs has been referred to as traditionalism, and traditionalism is important to consider when delivering resources. For example, Indigenous (First Nations) women from southern Ontario expressed their preference for online cancer resources as well as contact information for traditional healers, local physicians, and cancer societies (Hoffman-Goetz & Friedman, 2007).

Coe et al. (2004) examined disease risk factors, such as smoking, obesity, and alcohol consumption, among Hopi (Arizona Tribe, USA) women and found that higher levels of traditionalism, of which language is an important component, were associated with higher levels of disease protective behaviors. Gonzales et al. (2012) examined the effect of Indigenous language use on rates of colorectal cancer screening among the Hopi. While their findings failed to find evidence to support the use of Indigenous language as a barrier, the researchers noted that in this group (the Hopi), there were high levels of traditionalism with Indigenous language often acquired simultaneously with English, and this multilingualism may have facilitated understanding of English-language based health materials pertaining to the importance of cancer screening (Gonzales et al., 2012).

While the use of Indigenous language varies among Native Nations, its use certainly interacts with health behaviors, thus making it imperative to "disentangle the effects of language on health risks" (Woloshin et al., 1997). Health care professionals working with Indigenous populations agreed that there are language and cultural barriers in the provision of care, since "medical language and health concepts … derive from the dominant culture and often compete with Indigenous perspectives and understandings of health" (Lambert et al., 2014, p. 5). However, attempts to date have been less than clear in defining the role of Indigenous language in cancer disparities or whether language can or should be examined independently of other features of traditionalism. In a study comparing experiences of cancer patients and survivors among urban and rural Indigenous populations, Itty et al. (2014) found barriers of miscommunication and misunderstandings by both groups in their communication with providers. Some of these barriers resulted from language differences as well as providers' lack of understanding of Indigenous culture.

In their review, Gonzales et al. (2012) described the inconsistent findings of studies examining language use and preventative health behaviors with some studies failing to find significant relationships with Indigenous language use or cultural identification (Coe et al., 2004, 2007; Giuliano et al., 1998; Schumacher et al., 2008; Solomon & Gottlieb, 1999). They also point out, however, that "[s]tudies across many different Native Nations have commonly argued that themes, values, and symbols associated with tribal cultures can function as important resources for encouraging health knowledge and healthy behaviors, including behaviors relevant to cancer screening" (Gonzales et al., 2012, p. 796). Given these inconsistencies in the literature, it is clear that much still needs to be learned about the role that the use of Indigenous language can play in health interventions and health literacy education (Strickland et al., 1996, 1999; Hodge et al., 1996).

Of course, interventions and the improvement of heath literacy among Indigenous language speaking populations is more than simply translating health information. It has been noted that Indigenous languages are intertwined with culture and traditions that are not apparent to majority populations or health care providers. This is best understood by examining the efforts by Yost et al. (2017) to improve cancer literacy among Diné women through use of an intervention with an existing instrument, the Cancer Health Literacy Measure—Breast and Cervical Cancer. The development of an effective intervention required forward-translation (English to Diné) and backward-translation (Diné to English) by independent Diné language experts and a rigorous iterative process of review and cultural adaptation to capture beliefs about cancer unique to Diné culture. Some questions were modified in both English and Diné to ensure that the *intent* of the question was properly conveyed given the different interpretations of meaning by Diné people (Yost et al., 2017). This new instrument incorporated "attitudes, beliefs, knowledge, and emotions" of Diné culture that will help improve access and health literacy among the Diné women and provide for better validity and reliability of the data collected.

It is important to note that methods used with one population may not have the same outcomes with other populations since language-based solutions to health literacy in Indigenous populations are not "one-size-fits-all." To date, the work of Yost et al. (2017) appears to be the method most transferable among many different Indigenous populations given its focus on unique aspects of language and culture. An effective translation is one that incorporates semantic, idiomatic, technical, and conceptual equivalence specifically targeted toward the specific language and Indigenous population. Through this improved method of health literacy and information translation, the meaning and purpose of cancer prevention actions, screenings, and health care provision can be better communicated to Indigenous populations.

4 Historical Context Needed for Working with Indigenous Languages in Health Literacy and Cancer Prevention Efforts

Indigenous languages have suffered greatly over the past 200 years, largely due to assimilationist policies once instituted by the United States and State governments, with the intent to "Kill the Indian, and save the man," as stated by Brigadier General Richard Henry Pratt, founder of the Carlisle Indian Industrial School (Pratt, 1973). Beginning in 1879, the US governments used education as a means of assimilating Native American children, by replacing their Indigenous languages with English. According to a National Public Radio broadcast, at one point, the United States alone operated as many as 100 boarding schools tasked with transforming Indigenous children into "productive" members of American society (Bear, 2008). These federal and state boarding schools forbade the use of Indigenous languages, which led to a drastic decline in the number of fluent Indigenous language speakers. According to the Historic American Building Survey, the oldest orphanage-turned residential boarding school was in New York State, named the Thomas Indian School, on the Cattaraugus Territory of the Seneca Nation and operated from 1898 until it closed in 1956 (U.S. Department of the Interior, n.d.; Haynes et al., 2024).

Due to devastating federal assimilationist educational policies, which condemned the use of Indigenous languages, Native Nations currently have a small number of fluent first-language speakers. However, many Nations continue to conduct ceremonies in their Indigenous language and never ceased, despite government attempts to eradicate their culture. In addition, many community leaders have always taught or shared the importance of language continuance. Partnerships that embrace continued empowerment of health literacy between Native Nations, cancer centers, and institutions of higher education is imperative for survival and growth.

5 QI Process: Working with Elders, First-Language Speakers, and Urban Communities

These meetings began with introductions followed by the sharing of the English version of cancer prevention materials and purposes of outreach. The team consisted of cancer center program assistants, a project lead, and summer interns. This collective team sought feedback, dialogue, and conversation from Indigenous elders and first-language speakers and urban-based community members. The conversations and outreach materials were guided by findings from a literature review on best methods for cancer prevention, and results were discussed with both the cancer center team and student teams at the collaborating university's Native American studies program.

The outreach materials were then revised by incorporating the knowledge gained from community-based Indigenous translations with elders and first-language speakers into Indigenous-adapted versions. This work was led by the cancer center's creative services team. Conversations between the "in the field" team and creative services team members also occurred where there was further sharing of the meanings of Indigenous words and translations. It was often the case that there was not an Indigenous word for certain English words and then optimal Indigenous words were used to describe what the English words had intended. The products were then re-shared with elders and first-language speakers to ensure proper translations and readability. Finally, agreed upon materials were brought back to the creative services team for final revisions (e.g., see Appendices A, B, and outreach material in Appendix C created after community meetings described above).

Prior to dissemination, feedback and gathering of multiple perspective is critical to a successful QI process. In order to accomplish this task, adapted materials were brought back to urban community members for final review. The use of virtual platforms including ZOOM and Microsoft's TEAMS allowed the QI team to interact effectively and the collective data received assisted us in setting goals, viewing progress, and exploring new pathways. Given the time frame of this QI project during a global pandemic and the need for social distancing, the use of virtual QI roundtables was deemed the most effective and safe approach. The virtual round tables were comparable to talking circles, a traditional format of communication among Indigenous populations. According to Boyd et al. (2021), talking circles can be used to discuss cancer-related knowledge via traditional Indigenous stories. As a QI project, where non-research was hosted outside of territories, reservations, and reserves, there was not an IRB protocol.

Overall, there were 16 community members, with the majority identifying as Black, Indigenous, or People of Color (BIPOC). Among participants, 10 were male, 2 identified as female, and 4 elected not to identify. Eleven of the participants were between the ages of 20–31, and five participants elected not to disclose their age. Materials were brought back for urban community review to gather perspectives on dissemination, applicability, and overall material improvement.

6 QI Community Feedback

Respondents felt that adapted materials would be supported by their respective health and community-based centers, and it was recommended that materials be disseminated immediately, strategically, and often. One member shared, *"Having a marketing campaign is important … I think it is important to have relevant materials … but I think a campaign would be what would impact care. It all needs to be wrapped up in a campaign that would reach out and get people's attention. When I say campaign, I mean a series of events or announcements and a distribution of materials … a promotion over time. Reach out to health centers and schools."* Respondents also shared that they enjoyed the informative approach to the material and that Indigenous language use was appealing with potential to improve the chances of it being read by BIPOC populations. This was exemplified by multiple community members who shared, *"... Adapted materials ... make me more curious and inquisitive"; "The materials will be useful because they comprise of diverse language and it makes it more inclusive"* and *"... adapted materials look appealing and informative"; "it's catchy and with the kind of information on it, it will insinuate questions and create curiosity."* However, members also encouraged more Indigenous-specific cancer statistics and the use of community-friendly language. Ultimately, the project's goal was to create culturally attuned cancer prevention materials that are ready for outreach, real-time distribution, dissemination, and immediate clinical setting use. This was positively reflected by one member who shared, *"These materials will improve patient care ... absolutely ... this is really going to serve a long away in (urban) health care services."*

7 Limitations and Future Directions

One potential limitation of the virtual roundtables was that the audience was BIPOC, with non-Indigenous lenses providing feedback on Indigenous materials. This project was also not hosted on a reservation, reserve, or territory-based setting. Thus, findings may not be fully translatable to a reservation/reserve/territory perspective. Findings also do not generalize to all tribes, bands, and communities. However, materials provide important foundational translational lessons. Collectively, we found the process, voice, and community input from a multicultural perspective to be beneficial. Future steps include further investigations of the importance of health literacy to cancer prevention and screening in Indigenous populations, i.e., research beyond mere QI projects. Future research can be structured using research methods and Indigenous theory to test the effectiveness of such marketing campaigns on behavioral change with regard to cancer screenings and prevention efforts. As professionals, we have a universal duty "to apply what we know at any given time to all people" (Freeman, 2004, p. 77). Simply put, if there are ways we can achieve longevity in everyday lives, it is our mission to deliver the message in the best way possible, including through material translations. Everyone has the right to understand how to prevent cancer by maintaining a healthy diet, exercising, and living a healthy lifestyle. If we continue to be culturally aware and open-minded about our differences, health care facilities can work toward equity and improved care across the cancer care continuum.

Acknowledgments Onöndowa'ga and Indigenous First-Language Speakers; Native American Community Services (Buffalo, NY); Roswell Park Department of Education; Roswell Park Creative Services; Roswell Park Center for Indigenous Cancer Services. Authors are from diverse tribal and band affiliations along with non-Indigenous allies. Nations included: Onondowahgah (Seneca), Tuscarora, Mohawk, Anishinaabe, Fond Du Lac and Bad River Band of Lake Superior Chippewa, Six Nations-Onondaga, and Diné/Navajo Nations.

This work was supported by Roswell Park Comprehensive Cancer Center and a National Cancer Institute (NCI) grant, P30CA016056; the Bristol Meyers Squibb Foundation; and Roswell Park's Department of Indigenous Cancer Health and Indigenous & Rural Patient Navigation Program.

Appendix A

ROSWELL PARK COMPREHENSIVE CANCER CENTER

Ohä:tgi' Ye'dó'sageh *Info Sheet*
(Breast Cancer)

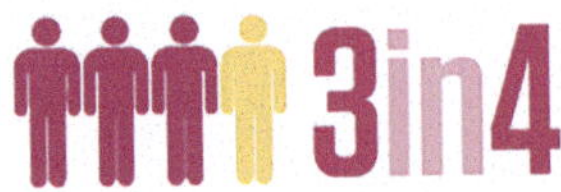

women with breast cancer have no family history of the disease and were **not** high risk

3 REASONS
TO GET YOUR MAMMOGRAM AT ROSWELL PARK

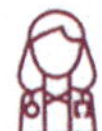

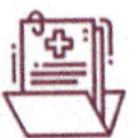

- **Our Expertise** with performing and reading advanced breast imaging including 3D mammography, ultrasound and MRI.
- **Convenience** of free, on-site parking, evening hours and express appointments that may take less than 30 minutes.
- **Comprehensive care** from trusted providers should you require biopsy or further treatment.

Call us to schedule your screening today: 1-800-ROSWELL (1-800-767-9355).

WHO GETS Ohä:tgi' Ye'dó'sageh (BREAST CANCER)?

Anyone can get breast cancer, and most women who develop breast cancer have no known risk factors. That's why ALL women must be screened regularly for breast cancer. The causes remain unclear, but some factors place you at **high risk** for the disease, such as:

- A family history of breast cancer among your parents, siblings or at least two other close relatives
- A personal or family history of ovarian cancer
- Multiple cancers within your family
- A relative diagnosed with breast cancer before menopause
- A known gene mutation, such as BRCA1, BRCA2, TP53, or PTEN in your family
- An abnormal breast biopsy
- Prior radiation to the chest

ARE YOU AT HIGH RISK FOR Ohä:tgi' Ye'dó'sageh (BREAST CANCER)?

Roswell Park's **Breast Cancer Risk Assessment and Prevention Program** provides a comprehensive assessment, surveillance exams and imaging, risk reduction and prevention options, genetic counseling and testing and access to clinical trials focused on prevention.

NOT SURE? Call 1-800-ROSWELL (1-800-767-9355) or take our assessment quiz at: Forms.RoswellPark.org/highrisk-breast

WHERE WE STAND

Roswell Park recommends women **begin annual mammography screening at age 40,** because this guidance saves the most lives. Talk to your healthcare provider about whether your personal risk factors warrant earlier or enhanced screening.

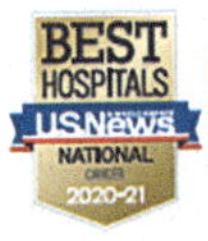

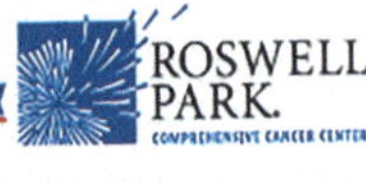

1-800-ROSWELL (1-800-767-9355) | RoswellPark.org

Appendix B

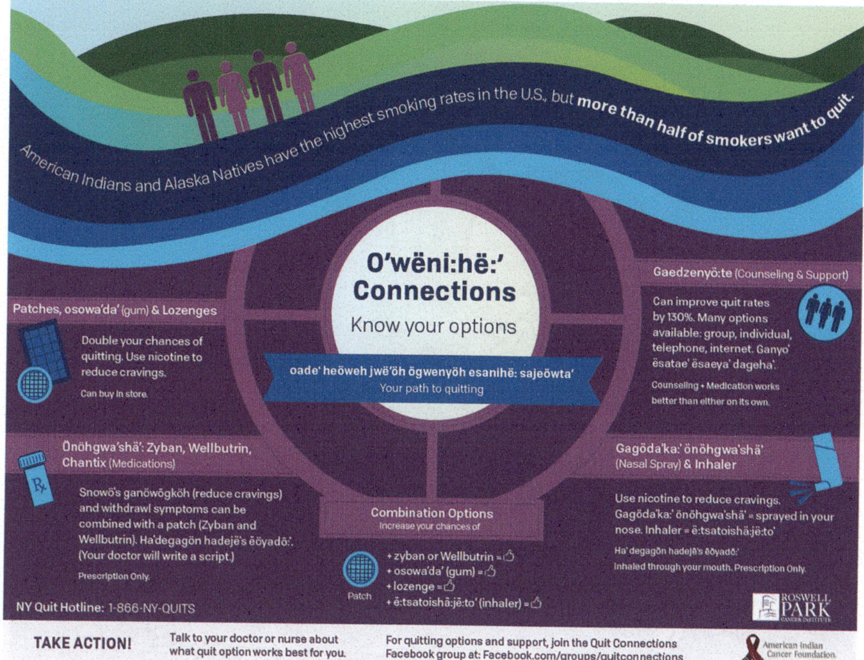
American Indians and Alaska Natives have the highest smoking rates in the U.S., but more than half of smokers want to quit.
O'wëni:hë:'
Connections
Know your options
oade' heöweh jwë'öh ögwenyöh esanihë: sajeöwta'
Your path to quitting
Patches, osowa'da' (gum) & Lozenges
Double your chances of quitting. Use nicotine to reduce cravings.
Can buy in store.
Önöhgwa'shä': Zyban, Wellbutrin, Chantix (Medications)
Snowö's ganöwögköh (reduce cravings) and withdrawl symptoms can be combined with a patch (Zyban and Wellbutrin). Ha'degagön hadejë's ëöyadö:'. (Your doctor will write a script.)
Prescription Only.
Gaedzenyö:te (Counseling & Support)
Can improve quit rates by 130%. Many options available: group, individual, telephone, internet. Ganyo' ësatae' ësaeya' dageha'.
Counseling + Medication works better than either on its own.
Gagöda'ka:' önöhgwa'shä' (Nasal Spray) & Inhaler
Use nicotine to reduce cravings. Gagöda'ka:' önöhgwa'shä' = sprayed in your nose. Inhaler = ë:tsatoishä:jë:to'
Ha' degagön hadejë's ëöyadö:'
Inhaled through your mouth. Prescription Only.
Combination Options
Increase your chances of
Patch
+ zyban or Wellbutrin =
+ osowa'da' (gum) =
+ lozenge =
+ ë:tsatoishä:jë:to' (inhaler) =
NY Quit Hotline: 1-866-NY-QUITS
ROSWELL PARK
TAKE ACTION!
Talk to your doctor or nurse about what quit option works best for you.
For quitting options and support, join the Quit Connections Facebook group at: Facebook.com/groups/quitconnections
American Indian Cancer Foundation

Appendix C

EXERCISE
Daily physical activity may reduce the likelihood of developing colorectal cancer.
SCREENING
Screening identifies potential cancer at earlier stages and may improve lifespan. CICR supports the U.S. Prevention Services Task Force recommendation of screening all adults for colorectal cancer **starting at age 45** when possible.
DIET
Eating foods directly of the land has an immediate impact on the health of your colon.
Your decisions influence your chances of developing cancer.
INDIGENOUS LIFEWAYS CAN HELP PREVENT COLORECTAL CANCER.
For more information about colorectal cancer screening please contact your primary care office, or call the Center For Indigenous Cancer Research (CICR) patient navigation program at
1-888-RPGUIDE (1-888-774-8433)
LIKE US ON FACEBOOK
ROSWELL PARK
VISIT US ONLINE

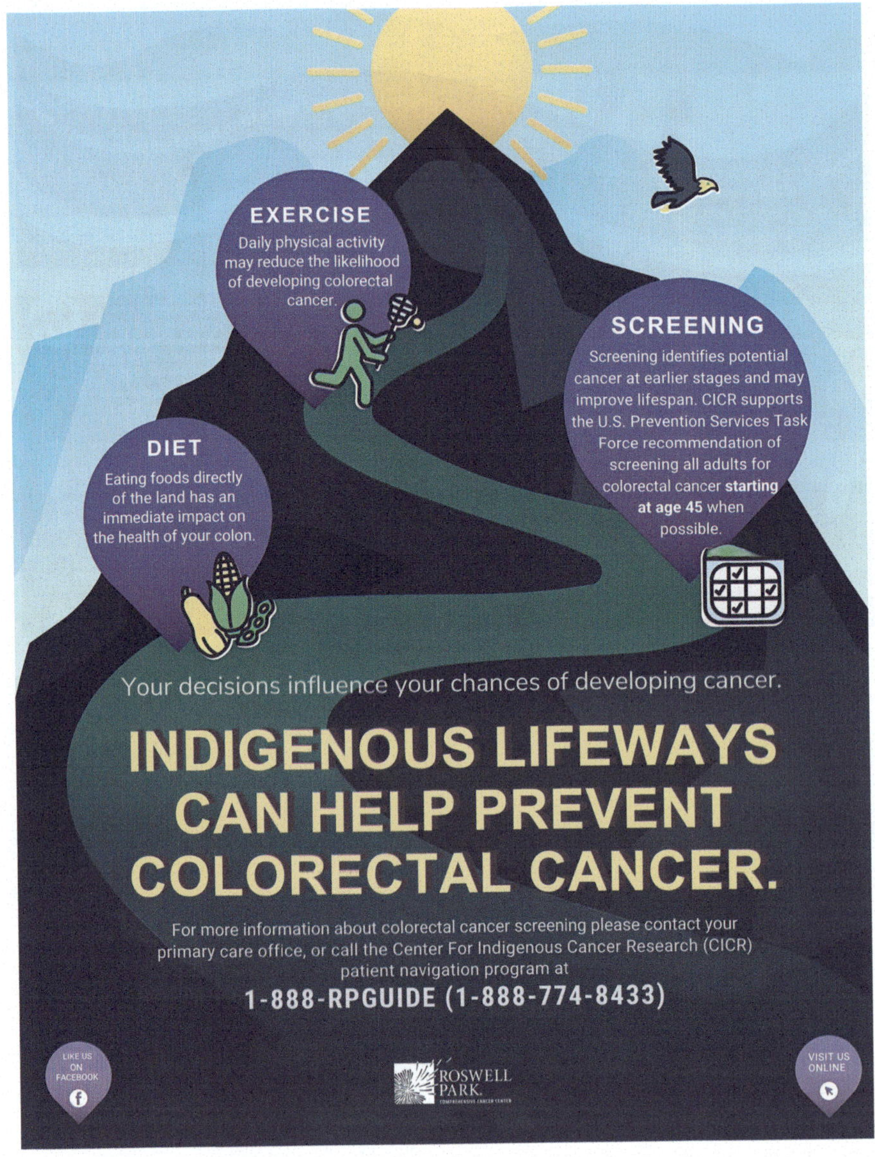

References

Bear, C. (2008, May 12). *American Indian boarding schools haunt many* (radio broadcast, National Public Radio's Morning Edition).

Beyea, S. C., & Nicoll, L. H. (1998). Is it research or quality improvement? *AORN Journal, 68*(1), 117–119. https://doi.org/10.1016/S0001-2092(06)62732-4

Boyd, A. D., Song, X., & Furgal, C. M. (2021). A systematic literature review of cancer communication with indigenous populations in Canada and the United States. *Journal of Cancer Education, 36*(2), 310–324. https://doi.org/10.1007/s13187-019-01630-2

Brega, A. G., Pratte, K. A., Jiang, L., Mitchell, C. M., Stotz, S. A., LoudHawk-Hedgepeth, C., Morse, B. D., Noe, T., Moore, K. R., & Beals, J. (2013). Impact of targeted health promotion on cardiovascular knowledge among American Indians and Alaska Natives. *Health Education Research, 28*(3), 437–449. https://doi.org/10.1093/her/cyt054

Coe, K., Attakai, A., Papenfuss, M., Giuliano, A., Martin, L., & Nuvayestewa, L. (2004). Traditionalism and its relationship to disease risk and protective behaviors of women living on the Hopi reservation. *Health Care for Women International, 25*(5), 391–410. https://doi.org/10.1080/07399330490438314

Coe, K., Martin, L., Nuvayestewa, L., Attakai, A., Papenfuss, M., de Zapien, J. G., Seymour, S. S., Hunter, J., & Giuliano, A. (2007). Predictors of Pap test use among women living on the Hopi reservation. *Health Care for Women International, 28*(9), 764–781. https://doi.org/10.1080/07399330701562956

Espey, D. K., Wu, X. C., Swan, J., Wiggins, C., Jim, M. A., Ward, E., Wingo, P. A., Howe, H. L., Ries, L. A. G., Miller, B. A., Jemal, A., Ahmed, F., Cobb, N., Kaur, J. S., & Edwards, B. K. (2007). Annual report to the nation on the status of cancer, 1975–2004, featuring cancer in American Indians and Alaska Natives. *Cancer, 110*(10), 2119–2152. https://doi.org/10.1002/cncr.23044

Freeman, H. P. (2004). Poverty, culture, and social injustice: Determinants of cancer disparities. *CA: A Cancer Journal for Clinicians, 54*(2), 72–77. https://doi.org/10.3322/canjclin.54.2.72

Giuliano, A., Papenfuss, M., de Guernsey de Zapien, J., Tilousi, S., & Nuvayestewa, L. (1998). Breast cancer screening among southwest American Indian women living on-reservation. *Preventive Medicine, 27*(1), 135–143. https://doi.org/10.1006/pmed.1997.0258

Gonzales, A. A., Garroutte, E., Ton, T. G. N., Goldberg, J., & Buchwald, D. (2012). Effect of tribal language use on colorectal cancer screening among American Indians. *Journal of Immigrant and Minority Health, 14*, 975–982. https://doi.org/10.1007/s10903-012-9598-2

Grady, C. (2015). Institutional review boards: Purpose and challenges. *Chest, 148*(5), 1148–1155.

Haring, R. C., Jim, M. A., Erwin, D., Kaur, J., Henry, W. A. E., Haring, M. L., & Seneca, D. S. (2018). Mortality disparities: A comparison with the Haudenosaunee in New York State. *Cancer Health Disparities, 2*. https://companyofscientists.com/index.php/chd/article/view/70

Haynes, H., McCarthy, T., Abrams, C., Lewis, M. E., & Haring, R. C. (2024). Revisiting one of the oldest orphanages, asylums, and Indigenous residential boarding schools: The Thomas Indian School at Seneca Nation. *International Journal of Environmental Research and Public Health, 21*(9), 1120. https://doi.org/10.3390/ijerph21091120

Hodge, F. S., Fredericks, L., & Rodriguez, B. (1996). American Indian women's talking circle. A cervical cancer screening and prevention project. *Cancer, 78*(7 Suppl), 1592–1597. https://doi.org/10.1002/(SICI)1097-0142(19961001)78:7+<1592::AID-CNCR13>3.0.CO;2-0

Hoffman-Goetz, L., & Friedman, D. B. (2007). A qualitative study of Canadian Aboriginal women's beliefs about "credible" cancer information on the Internet. *Journal of Cancer Education, 22*, 124–128. https://doi.org/10.1007/BF03174361

Itty, T. L., Hodge, F. S., & Martinez, F. (2014). Shared and unshared barriers to cancer symptom management among urban and rural American Indians. *The Journal of Rural Health, 30*(2), 206–213. https://doi.org/10.1111/jrh.12045

Jones, D., Lyle, D., McAllister, L., Randall, S., Dyson, R., White, D., Smith, A., Hampton, D., Goldsworthy, M., & Rowe, A. (2020). The case for integrated health and community literacy to achieve transformational community engagement and improved health outcomes: An inclusive approach to addressing rural and remote health inequities and community healthcare expectations. *Primary Health Care Research & Development, 21*, e57. https://doi.org/10.1017/S1463423620000481

Keleher, H., & Hagger, V. (2007). Health literacy in primary health care. Special issue on "comparative approaches to primary health care: key lessons for Australia's primary health care policy-making". *Australian Journal of Primary Health, 13*, 24–30. https://search.informit.org/doi/10.3316/informit.089019520306287

Kutner, M., Greenberg, E., Jin, Y., Paulsen, C., & White, S. (2006). The health literacy of America's adults: Results from the 2003 National Assessment of Adult Literacy (NCES 2006–483). U.S. Department of Education, National Center for Education Statistics.

Lakhan, P., Askew, D., Harris, M. F., Kirk, C., & Hayman, N. (2017). Understanding health talk in an urban Aboriginal and Torres Strait Islander primary healthcare service: A cross-sectional study. *Australian Journal of Primary Health, 23*(4), 335–341. https://doi.org/10.1071/PY16162

Lambert, M., Luke, J., Downey, B., Crengle, S., Kelaher, M., Reid, S., & Smylie, J. (2014). Health literacy: Health professionals' understandings and their perceptions of barriers that Indigenous patients encounter. *BMC Health Services Research, 14*, 614. https://doi.org/10.1186/s12913-014-0614-1

Pratt, R. H. (1973). Official report of the nineteenth annual conference of charities and correction (1892), 46–59. Reprinted in Richard H. Pratt, "The advantages of mingling Indians with Whites," *Americanizing the American Indians: Writings by the "Friends of the Indian"* 1880–1900 (pp. 260–271). Harvard University Press.

Reinhardt, A. C., & Ray, L. N. (2003). Differentiating quality improvement from research. *Applied Nursing Research, 16*(1), 2–8. https://doi.org/10.1053/apnr.2003.59000

Roh, S., Burnette, C. E., Lee, Y. S., Jun, J. S., Lee, H. Y., & Lee, K. H. (2018). Breast cancer literacy and health beliefs related to breast cancer screening among American Indian women. *Social Work in Health Care, 57*(7), 465–482. https://doi.org/10.1080/00981389.2018.1455789

Rootman, I., & Gordon-El-Bihbety, D. (2008). *A vision for a health literate Canada: Report of the expert panel on health literacy*. Canadian Public Health Association.

Schumacher, M. C., Slattery, M. L., Lanier, A. P., Ma, K.-N., Edwards, S., Ferucci, E. D., & Tom-Orme, L. (2008). Prevalence and predictors of cancer screening among American Indian and Alaska native people: The EARTH study. *Cancer Causes & Control, 19*(7), 725–737. https://doi.org/10.1007/s10552-008-9135-8

Smith, J. A., Merlino, A., Christie, B., Adams, M., Bonson, J., Osborne, R., Judd, B., Drummond, M., Aanundsen, D., & Fleay, J. (2020). 'Dudes are meant to be tough as nails': The complex nexus between masculinities, culture and health literacy from the perspective of young Aboriginal and Torres Strait Islander males – Implications for policy and practice. *American Journal of Men's Health, 14*(3). https://doi.org/10.1177/1557988320936121

Solomon, T. G., & Gottlieb, N. H. (1999). Measures of American Indian traditionality and its relationship to cervical cancer screening. *Health Care for Women International, 20*(5), 493–504. https://doi.org/10.1080/073993399245584

Strickland, C. J., Chrisman, N. J., Yallup, M., Powell, K., & Squeoch, M. D. (1996). Walking the journey of womanhood: Yakama Indian women and Papanicolaou (Pap) test screening. *Public Health Nursing, 13*(2), 141–150. https://doi.org/10.1111/j.1525-1446.1996.tb00232.x

Strickland, C. J., Squeoch, M. D., & Chrisman, N. J. (1999). Health promotion in cervical cancer prevention among the Yakama Indian women of the Wa'Shat Longhouse. *Journal of Transcultural Nursing, 10*(3), 190–196. https://doi.org/10.1177/104365969901000309

Thewes, B., McCaffery, K., Davis, E., & Garvey, G. (2018). Insufficient evidence on health literacy amongst Indigenous people with cancer: A systematic literature review. *Health Promotion International, 33*(2), 195–218. https://doi.org/10.1093/heapro/daw066

U.S. Department of the Interior. (n.d.). *Historic American buildings survey mid-Atlantic region*. National Park Service. HABS No. NY-6012.

Webkamigad, S., Warry, W., Blind, M., & Jacklin, K. (2020). An approach to improve dementia health literacy in Indigenous communities. *Journal of Cross-Cultural Gerontology, 35*(1), 69–83. https://doi.org/10.1007/s10823-019-09388-2

Woloshin, S., Schwartz, L. M., Katz, S. J., & Welch, H. G. (1997). Is language a barrier to the use of preventive services? *Journal of General Internal Medicine, 12*(8), 472–477. https://doi.org/10.1046/j.1525-1497.1997.00085.x

Yost, K. J., Bauer, M. C., Buki, L. P., Austin-Garrison, M., Garcia, L. V., Hughes, C. A., & Patten, C. A. (2017). Adapting a cancer literacy measure for use among Navajo women. *Journal of Transcultural Nursing, 28*(3), 278–285. https://doi.org/10.1177/1043659616628964

Health Communications Development and Dissemination for a Media Campaign in Support of Indigenous Health, Cancer Prevention, and Early Detection

Rodney C. Haring, Will Maybee, Josie Raphaelito, Jaiden Mitchell, Ana Yulaly Stahlman, and Paul Hage

Abstract Cancer and health-related community outreach and education efforts continually rely on health communications to reach and inform important target audiences. Community-based presentations, prevention messaging, and dissemination of cancer screening information to increase knowledge and preventative behaviors among Indigenous communities are critically important because cancer is one of the leading drivers of morbidity and mortality. As an exemplar, media-based health communication efforts led by community partners in a collaborative framework with a federally (USA) designated cancer center's Department of Indigenous Cancer Health, Community Outreach and Engagement program, and Health Communications Resource are shared. Communications were designed for Indigenous media networks and community-based film companies. Topics included health, cancer prevention, and cancer screening. The health communication model for dissemination of mass media creations involved film and media screenings, panel discussions, and influencer platforms integration; communications were preserved in the cancer center's Indigenous outreach and engagement digital repository. Evaluation efforts to improve the quality of health communication processes revealed the importance of coproducing films under the guidance of community advisory boards, and conducting surveys of knowledge, attitudes, and prevention and screening behaviors. These experiences highlight how organizations responsible for cancer care can create engaging stories and health messaging for Indigenous communities.

R. C. Haring (✉) · W. Maybee · J. Raphaelito · A. Y. Stahlman
Department of Indigenous Cancer Health, Roswell Park Comprehensive Cancer Center, Buffalo, NY, USA
e-mail: Rodney.Haring@RoswellPark.org

J. Mitchell
Dreamcatcher Studio, 160 School Rd Hogansburg, United States, NY, USA

P. Hage
Health Communications Resource, Roswell Park Comprehensive Cancer Center, Buffalo, NY, USA

R. C. Haring (ed.), *Indigenous Genetics, Biobanking, Chemistry, and Cancer Research*, Cancer Health Disparities, https://doi.org/10.1007/978-3-032-17296-9_8

Keywords Cancer · Health communications · Media · Mass communications · Dissemination · Indigenous knowledge · Indigenous · Native American · First Nations · Native Hawaiian · Alaska Native · Inuit · Metis · BIPOC · Cancer prevention · Education · STEM · STEAM · Science · Arts · Film · Social media · Influencers · Storytelling · Health messaging · Visibility

1 Introduction

Health communications teams can support cancer prevention and early detection efforts by creating engaging mass media platforms for storytelling and messaging that increase the visibility of underserved populations, raise awareness, promote education, share important health data, and encourage behavior changes to reduce cancer risk. The field of health communications also can play an instrumental role in efforts to reduce cancer health disparities (Haring et al., 2018) by developing culturally conducive messages, materials, and programs that resonate widely with politically delineated entities such as sovereign Native Nations along with Black (https://www.nlm.nih.gov/nativevoices/timeline/427.html), Indigenous (urban, reservation, reserve), and Peoples of Color (BIPOC) communities.

Health communications within the fields of cancer sciences convey many aspects of the Science, Technology, Engineering, and Math or STEM fields. In many cancer care centers that carry out research, messaging can be developed around various scientific projects, including qualitative research and quantitative science such as mixed-methods research and basic, translational, and clinical science. The “S” in STEM is well represented in cancer studies—notable examples are genetic discoveries in cancer that have translated into improved screening and care procedures for targeted populations. The “S” in STEM is also represented in cancer center education departments and programs. For example, Roswell Park Comprehensive Cancer Center’s Department of Indigenous Cancer Health has received collaborative education awards for STEM work in partnership with Indigenous Nations and the U.S. National Institutes of Health, in support of the Akwesasne Research Centers for Health (ARCH) program (NIH 5S06GM142118-03). Roswell Park’s technology transfer and intellectual property in science division represents the “T” in areas of STEM science. Engineering in science can be found throughout the medical campus via collaborative efforts in support of the functioning and maintenance of STEM-based facilities and laboratories. Lastly, the “M” in STEM science at many National Cancer Institute (NCI)-designated cancer centers and academic medical centers is represented by robust statistical programs that support cancer-focused projects. For example, Roswell Park hosts a Biostatistics and Statistical Genomics Shared Resource whose team consists of cancer-focused mathematicians, statisticians, and epidemiologists.

Recently, Roswell Park's Department of Indigenous Cancer Health created a position based on STEAM (STEM plus the Arts) principles that focuses on the art of media production, film, and digital health communications. The intern reflected on her efforts by sharing:

> In the Department for Indigenous Cancer Health as a STEAM intern I have been focusing on collaborative efforts that integrate media, communications, and the performing arts. My work aims to decrease cancer and co-occurring health disparities within Indigenous communities in both rural and urban settings. My experience has had interdisciplinary approaches; including research, media, creative collaborative not only within the Haudenosaunee Confederacy but with other tribes on Turtle Island. My favorite part of my internship is having the creative freedom to [produce] culturally responsive solutions that promote awareness, prevention, and improved health outcomes.
>
> —Personal communication, Ana Yulaly Stahlman, March 11, 2025

In total, many cancer centers and academic medical centers have programs that are well-rounded in terms of basic, translational, and clinical research, patient care, and education-based activities that advance STEM fields. STEM has proven useful as a conceptual organizing principle, and broadening this to STEAM—Science, Technology, Engineering, Art, and Mathematics—can be beneficial in certain contexts (Bequette & Bequette, 2012). This chapter describes the authors' efforts to enhance science-based innovations in "art" at a comprehensive cancer center within the Health Communications Resource (HCR) (Hage & Haring 2023) in collaboration with the Department of Indigenous Cancer Health and the Community Outreach and Engagement program. Examples blend cancer science and art focused on film, health media, public service announcements, short video productions for social media (e.g., horizontal 1-minute shorts for Facebook, Instagram, TikTok), and longer health documentaries.

2 Translating Data to Outreach Through Digital Media

Cancer health-related community outreach and education efforts progressively rely on digital media creations to reach and inform important target audiences. Strong, collaborative, and bidirectional relationships are the foundation for effective outreach and health communications. Infrastructures conducive to building and sustaining community trust and collaboration are also imperative for outreach, health data sharing, and dissemination. Community outreach and engagement are fundamental components of cancer health initiatives. According to Shin et al. (2020), "The definition of community health outreach is a temporary, mobile project that involves the collaboration of a community to undertake its purposeful health intervention of reaching a population facing health risks." Oftentimes, Indigenous outreach expands on these criteria. This may include outreach models that are driven by direction from Community Advisory Boards (CABs). CABs incorporated into health communications development and dissemination can help identify areas of need among community groups and guide responsible health data sharing and dissemination.

Overall, community outreach and engagement in the cancer center context can facilitate cross-collaborative efforts between academic teams and tribal outreach media teams. Collaborative efforts may also include academic or cancer center government affairs teams and tribal government offices. Outreach with Indigenous governments often requires a multilevel, systematic approach, and it is useful to allocate time for this. Traditional approaches to couple health communications and digital media may also include discussions at national and international scientific meetings, presentations in Indigenous communities, and information sharing through newsletters, peer-reviewed publications, and other community resources.

Digital health communications are widely recognized as an important tool among communication researchers, especially when an emotional connection can be made with audiences so that there is enhanced motivation for behavioral change. This chapter highlights the process by which we developed, shared, and archived digital media for the Multi-Channel Communication Campaigns for Improvements in Cancer Education and Outcomes (MICEO) in Underserved Populations program. This work involved expanding on innovative means of health communications and braiding arts, culture, and Indigenous translations into science through a systematic process.

It is always best to understand and incorporate the target audience's cultural values, beliefs, identity, and traditions wherever possible within the filmmaking process to enhance acceptance of health information or behavior change desired by the producers (Kreuter & McClure, 2004). Filmmakers have many tools and elements to consider when creating health-media for specific populations. These elements include decisions about film locations, actor or interviewee attire, music, and other cultural elements within the production. By authentically representing and partnering with those in the community, health communications can foster a greater sense of familiarity, respect, and acceptance among viewers.

To address cancer disparities among Indigenous communities, Roswell Park launched a FilmsFilms for Indigenous Cancer Health (FICH) series, in which health communication films were created with social media influencers and Indigenous icons for use on social media and in community-based health centers (e.g., Indigenous-related health television networks, Indigenous social media channels). Production was carried out through the collaborative effort of Roswell Park's Health Communications Resource (HCR), a shared resource that houses a full-service video and media production center and has experience in creating health communications for local, regional, national, and international audiences. HCR helps investigators, institutions, and community health advocates educate the public about important health-related matters and promote health services. The HCR's main area of focus is on understanding the many determinants that influence health behaviors and application of that knowledge to reduce the burden of illness and chronic disease through the creation of effective, salient, and emotive media.

Productions described here integrated community-based practices, prevention messaging, and cancer screening information with the aim of increasing knowledge, intent, and behaviors among Indigenous members and communities. The work was accomplished by collaborative efforts from the HCR and Indigenous media networks and community-based film companies. Indigenous icons and influencers were also actively involved in content creation and messaging, which represented an additional layer to the community engagement and co-development process.

One example of integration during the production and editing of a project is where producers took extra steps to record and film an authentic Indigenous flute player from the community, instead of using a readily available stock music selection in the soundtrack. The viewing audience was cognizant and appreciative of this detail, which garnered more positive feelings toward the production. Another example of this approach was the intentional use of cultural representations and specific visual elements such as colors, symbolism, and other aesthetic choices by the producers.

Kreuter and McClure identified several approaches commonly used to achieve cultural appropriateness in health communication programs, and these were categorized as peripheral, evidential, linguistic, and sociocultural mechanisms (Kreuter & McClure, 2004). *Peripheral* approaches are those that enhance health communications by presenting content in ways that are appealing to target audiences, through use of certain colors, images, fonts, or pictures relevant to the group. *Evidential* and *linguistic* approaches incorporate health impact data and native language elements, respectively. *Sociocultural* approaches present content grounded in the context of the direct experiences of the targeted audience. The FICH films have many visual elements that are specific to Indigenous ways of life and represented during the production process. By prioritizing cultural authenticity through collaborative efforts and participatory methods, filmmakers can create impactful narratives that not only educate but also empower communities to actively engage in their health journeys.

One long-term goal of the work was integration toward continuance and collaboration with the community outreach and engagement (COE) teams at Roswell Park Comprehensive Cancer Center and the cancer center's Department of Indigenous Cancer Health, which houses a community outreach team that leads outreach efforts focused on media-to-media relationships between NCI-designated cancer center areas and Native Nations along with Indigenous urban, suburban, and rural areas (e.g., collaborations with Fred Hutch Cancer Center). The COE and the Indigenous outreach team continue to build sustainable integration pathways into both cancer center and Indigenous services delivery systems for ongoing dissemination of video work, health messaging about evidence-based cancer education, screening, and treatment services, and information on open clinical trials. Results have increased community-based outreach through health messaging. Gary Farmer, who collaborated on the project, said:

> I think it's really important that I continue to inform, educate and socialize people; keeping them abreast of things they're not necessarily thinking about. I'm glad I have some time to be a thinker and to move forward with stories that I think are vital to our healthy future.
>
> —Gary Farmer, Actor, Musician, Founding Director of the Aboriginal Voices Radio Network (Cayuga/Haudenosaunee, Six Nations of the Grand River)

3 Dissemination: Theory and Indigenous Philosophical Underpinnings

A recent publication on narrative communication theory suggests the "positioning of narrative practices to position theory" (Bamberg, 2024), which coincides with Fisher's Narrative Paradigm theory (Fisher, 1984, 1987) that stated humans are natural storytellers and all meaningful communication occurs by way of stories. In practice, narrative therapy, emerging from New Zealand, combined these theoretical concepts into counseling, therapy, and social work (White & Epston, 1990). Early antecedents to narrative therapy and narrative communication theory were the use of storytelling by Indigenous peoples across the world to document history, ways of life, science, and origins. More recently, narrative therapy has been practiced with Indigenous populations, particularly in narrative medicine approaches to address historical trauma and promote culturally sensitive care (Haring, 2013). Overall, ancient practices of storytelling, modern day concepts of narrative communication, and practiced-based narrative therapy share many similarities, as exemplified by the blending of community knowledge and personal experiences with the goals of personal and societal growth.

The development and dissemination of cancer-focused media and overall storytelling to improve health in Indigenous communities, and more broadly BIPOC communities, can be highly effective when led by both Indigenous knowledge and Indigenous-driven processes that integrate Western-based media communication models. One example involves the Transportation-Imagery Model of Narrative Communication. This model states that narrative communication and persuasion occur because an individual is "transported" into the narrative world in an "integrated melding of attention, imagery, and storied events." Meaning that, according to this model, individuals are so absorbed into the story that they are less likely pose counterarguments and more likely to believe the story propositions, identify with the story, and connect with the characters, which ultimately can allow the perspectives to have a great influence on the beliefs of the viewer (Bequette & Bequette, 2012; Hinyard & Kreuter, 2007). Narrative forms of communication include entertainment, education, journalism, and storytelling, and narrative communication can be used to influence healthy cancer preventative behaviors. This approach may be especially helpful for eliminating cancer disparities within minority populations where there is often distrust (Hinyard & Kreuter, 2007). Narrative ways of knowing can include engaging stories, gripping drama, and historical accounts.

Thus, Indigenous models integrated with contemporary theory can be used to shape film and other health media, and this may lead to greater dissemination and uptake in communities through pathways of benefit linking back to Indigenous health care centers, community grassroots organizations, and Indigenous serving not-for-profits that are in the process of mobilizing community-based collaborations. Exemplars include documentary-shorts wrapped in Indigenous frameworks of the Transportation-Imagery Model and narrative communication theory, which effectively deliver outreach and prevention messaging and connect people to services such as cancer-focused patient navigation (Henry et al., 2024).

The *sociocultural* approach to health messaging and media production also weaves a group's cultural values, beliefs, and behaviors into the actual script and discussion. These are incorporated by either being narrated, spoken by the interviewees, or displayed visually through text and graphics. For example, when Roswell Park's HCR creates media for Indigenous communities, time-honored and revered principles are often incorporated into the films. Principles such as the "Good Mind" and "7 Generations" add authenticity, depth, and potentially resonate with the viewer on a more meaningful and profound level. This approach helps reinforce the health message and its potential saliency by recognizing a culture's unique philosophical and spiritual underpinnings and creates connections between health information and historical values that help guide and inspire communities.

Films provide critical footage for continued cancer prevention program development, and archived content can be used to enhance programming and dissemination of health messages through media sharing. An example of digital storage to dissemination is Roswell Park's hosting of the Native C.I.R.C.L.E. (Cancer Information Resources Center and Learning Exchange). In 2020, Roswell Park Comprehensive Cancer Center acquired rights to the Native C.I.R.C.L.E. (Garcia et al., 2017) and embedded the content into Roswell Park's Department of Indigenous Cancer Health. Videos produced through FICH are added to the Native C.I.R.C.L.E. database for archiving and potential future dissemination. Native C.I.R.C.L.E. in current form is a comprehensive, interactive, and continuously updated educational and research resource for lay communities, policymakers, and researchers. The content can be used to foster collaboration and dialogue among scientists, Indigenous Nations, comprehensive cancer centers, patient advocacy groups, and members of Indigenous communities across North American and beyond. Native C.I.R.C.L.E. significantly increases the dissemination of resource materials developed from prior research endeavors, provides a wealth of expertise for new community education efforts around cancer and health, and allows for the exchange of ideas necessary for culturally appropriate interventions.

Roswell Park has recently begun to create health communication films and dissemination products with social media influencers and Indigenous icons as an important means for reaching the people. Productions of this nature integrate community-based practice, prevention messaging, and screening information to increase knowledge, intent, and behaviors among Indigenous members and communities as these relate to cancer and the need for early screening. Several factors are critical for success, including the creation and delivery of documentary-style short films and other media using outlined narrative communications coproduced in collaboration with community members throughout the videography, production, and editing processes. Additionally, posting short films and accompanying trailers online through commonly utilized video websites is important for accessibility, as is social media integration and training to ensure the appropriate posting of links and photography on social media networks. Equally as important is the creation of more visibility or representation in health messaging for underserved populations such as Indigenous communities. Short films screened during campaign months linked to specific topics in cancer awareness and prevention (e.g., March is colorectal cancer awareness month) may be particularly helpful for targeting of the leading cancer health disparities within Indigenous populations. Importantly, these films can educate people on the optimal cancer screening process and provide guiding information and resources.

Short film screenings in Indigenous communities can support partnership building between health clinics and NCI-designated cancer centers as well as support active efforts by the health care industry to address issues like mistrust and requests for visibility within health communication resources. During these community gatherings, this is also an opportunity to highlight additional health resources, introduce Indigenous staff and allies to contacts for obtaining additional information, and discuss shared pathways to STEAM careers and student enhancement initiatives for Indigenous community members.

4 Evaluative Process

Evaluation of cancer health dissemination programs is key to understanding whether programs are meeting parameters set forth by tribes, native urban centers, and Indigenous organizations to ensure services are making a positive difference in people's lives. Tracking of participation at events and venues is useful for community screenings of short films, and monitoring of social network sites' posts related to the screening can be informative. Social media engagement analytics may be available, and it may be possible to see which advocacy organizations are using the documentary for screenings with Indigenous Nations' councils and other policy- or decision-makers. Ideally, the short films will be shared with Indigenous health care providers regionally, and discussions at national and international scales can encourage continued dissemination practices among their respective communities. Attendees at film screenings can also complete pre- and post-screening surveys to assess changes in knowledge and attitudes about the health communications product's ability to increase cancer prevention knowledge and screening behaviors.

Computational methods also can be applied to digital trace data associated with publicly posted web objects related to various online or social media platforms. Thus, methods should support the gathering and archiving of trace data, which include "likes," "comments," and "views," and these data can be used to produce informative reports that track engagement with elements of dissemination over time, enabling health communication teams to relate variations on dissemination patterns of user engagement. Altogether, the use of innovative multimedia and community-based techniques in dissemination can improve outreach and advocacy over time.

Lastly, program evaluations of health communication trends and quality improvement findings allow for further information sharing back to partnering communities as a form of partnership building and benefice. For example, videos produced with Haudenosaunee (People of the Longhouse) influencer leaders across the United States and Canada were provided back to Haudenosaunee Confederacy and Indigenous urban landscapes. Specifically, collaborators were provided an open forum to show the documentary shorts across Indigenous health care media platforms (regional networks, local health care waiting rooms, television networks, and Indigenous urban center media outlets). Films were also presented at Indigenous film festivals and regional and national conferences that host media tracts.

5 Conclusion

Development and dissemination of innovative media-based health communications are an important means for providing the public with up-to-date information on cancer prevention and screening, effective treatments and surgical advances, and posttreatment care, including palliative care and survivorship information. This is especially true for Indigenous Nations who have sovereign news outlets and a sovereign voice, where reports originate from within sovereign Nation media and are communicated to internal and external audiences.

The growth of social media and diversification of platforms can allow for improved outreach to BIPOC and culturally diverse areas such as rural regions and sovereign Indigenous Nations worldwide. Cancer and health information created with communities for communities is important. Involving prominent voices such as influencers is a promising way to reach new audiences and is expected to lead to continued dissemination of impactful health information that can prevent cancer, increase cancer screenings, and save lives.

For health care audiences, Indigenous communities, and the fields of communication, the next steps will include continued exploration of health communication advances to promote disease prevention literacy and effective dissemination techniques, evaluation of health promotion data and statistics to gauge effectiveness, and continued education on cultural differences and the need to embrace inclusive language to avoid stigmatizing practices. Advancement will no doubt continue at the intersection of cancer and health promotion and the creation of health documentaries and interactive media. Strategic plans from local to global scales should aim to provide clear, transparent, and historical truths within messages and test concepts with target audiences prior to wider dissemination. The use of evidence-based or practiced-based (in diverse communities) strategies to promote behavior change is paramount for effective health communications development and dissemination that will sustain the wellness of people today and future generations. Responsible data use matters!

Acknowledgments The authors are grateful for guidance from the Roswell Park Comprehensive Cancer Center Indigenous Community Advisory Board, Corinne Porter, MPH, Richard Satterwhite, James Kennedy, Michael Johnson, and Gary Farmer. Funding support: 3P30CA016056-46S1 Cancer Data Talks in AI/AN/Native Hawaiian and Indigenous Landscapes; 3P30CA016056-47S1 Films for Indigenous Cancer Health; and 5S06GM142118-03 Akwesasne Research Centers for Health (ARCH) program. Overall, this work was supported by Roswell Park Comprehensive Cancer Center and National Cancer Institute (NCI) grant, P30CA016056.

References

Bamberg, M. (2024). Positioning, narrative practices, and positioning theory. In M. B. McVee, L. Van Langenhove, C. H. Brock, & B. A. Christensen (Eds.), *The Routledge international handbook of positioning theory*. Routledge. https://doi.org/10.4324/9781003288305-3

Bequette, J. W., & Bequette, M. B. (2012). A place for art and design education in the STEM conversation. *Art Education, 65*(2), 40–47.

Fisher, W. R. (1984). Narration as a human communication paradigm: The case of public moral argument. *Communication Monographs, 51*(1), 1–22. https://doi.org/10.1080/03637758409390180

Fisher, W. R. (1987). *Human communication as narration: Toward a philosophy of reason, value, and action*. University of South Carolina Press.

Garcia, A., Baethke, L., & Kaur, J. S. (2017). Lessons learned from Native C.I.R.C.L.E., a culturally specific resource. *Journal of Cancer Education, 32*, 740–744. https://doi.org/10.1007/s13187-016-1001-x

Hage, P., & Haring, R. C. (2023, July). *Health communications resource videos*. https://vimeo.com/channels/healthcommunications

Haring, R. C. (2013). Chapter 13. Using narrative therapy with Native American recreational tobacco users. *Substance Use & Misuse, 48*(13), 1434–1437. https://doi.org/10.3109/10826084.2013.815024

Haring, R. C., Jim, M. A., Erwin, D., Kaur, J. S., Henry, W. A. E., Haring, M. L., & Seneca, D. S. (2018). Mortality disparities: A comparison with the Haudenosaunee in New York State. *Cancer Health Disparities, 2*, e1–e20. https://pmc.ncbi.nlm.nih.gov/articles/PMC6880943/

Henry, W. A. E., Haring, M., Redeye, C., Phearsdorf, R., Washburn, N., & Haring, R. C. (2024). Two-row Wampum: Indigenous cancer patient navigation. In G. Garvey (Ed.), *Indigenous and tribal peoples and cancer*. Springer. https://doi.org/10.1007/978-3-031-56806-0_4

Hinyard, L. J., & Kreuter, M. W. (2007). Using narrative communication as a tool for health behavior change: A conceptual, theoretical, and empirical overview. *Health Education & Behavior, 34*(5), 777–792.

Kreuter, M. W., & McClure, S. M. (2004). The role of culture in health communication. *Annual Review of Public Health, 25*, 439–455. https://doi.org/10.1146/annurev.publhealth.25.101802.123000

Native Voices. *Native peoples' concepts of health and illness* [website]. NIH. https://www.nlm.nih.gov/nativevoices/timeline/427.html

Shin, H. Y., Kim, K. Y., & Kang, P. (2020). Concept analysis of community health outreach. *BMC Health Services Research, 20*(1), 417. https://doi.org/10.1186/s12913-020-05266-7

White, M., & Epston, D. (1990). *Narrative means to therapeutic ends*. W. W. Norton.

Closing Narratives

The artwork exemplifies the Tree of Peace, a symbol in Haudenosaunee (Iroquois) teachings that represent unity, diplomacy, and the Great Law of Peace that binds the Haudenosaunee Nations together. Wrapped around the tree is a strand of DNA, representing humanity's connection to the Earth—biologically and spiritually. Within the DNA are elements of the Haudenosaunee Thanksgiving Address (Ganonyok), an expression of gratitude that honors all aspects of Creation, from the land and waters to the plants, animals, and cosmic realms. This integration suggests that reciprocity and respect for nature are fundamental to our existence, much like the genetic code itself. The art further expands on using sky dome imagery illustrating the relationship between Earth and Sky, while Celestial Trees symbolizing life and wisdom, and unifying all elements in harmony. The artwork conveys a powerful message that peace is not just an ideal but a natural law, reminding us of our duty to live in balance, understanding data in various forms that sustain life and the world around us.

R. C. Haring (ed.), *Indigenous Genetics, Biobanking, Chemistry, and Cancer Research*, Cancer Health Disparities, https://doi.org/10.1007/978-3-032-17296-9

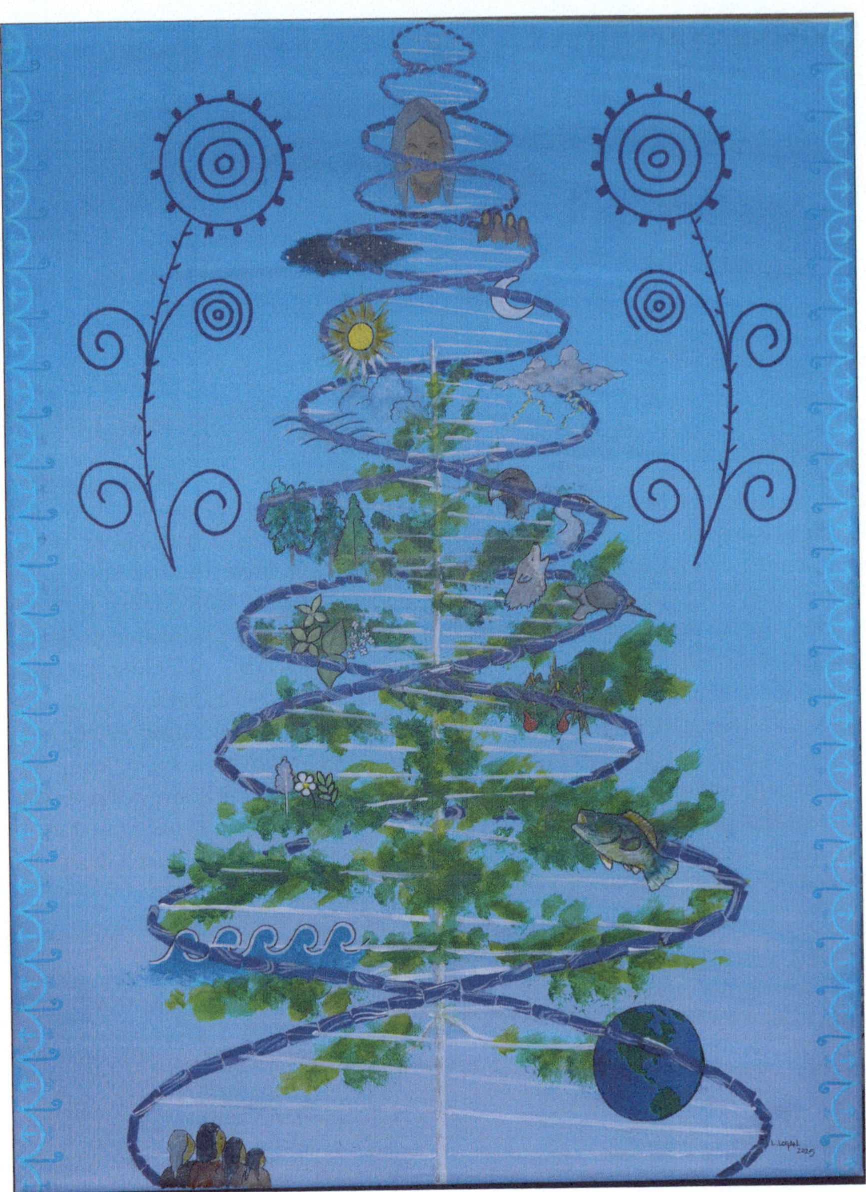

Artist Lyle Logan is an enrolled Seneca Nation member of the Deer clan. A cultural artisan, the majority of his work reflect aspects of Haudenosaunee culture and lifeways. Mr. Logan has been practicing his craft for 25 years and resides in Salamanca, New York, USA.

"We will gather information"—En'iakwariwarorokeh (the future matters of importance with be dealt with).

For the last 2000 years, the Great Law of Peace has been in the wampum. The wampum belts are our records of information. The symbols were our way of recording our stories. The wampum belts have a power to them and when you hold it, it turns on or activates the "recording" to be able to tell the story. It is important to gather all the information, good and bad, and accurately tell the truth of what happened in the past. An example is when the Great Law talks about when we were cannibals, and we did very bad things to each other. It is included so we don't repeat the bad history again. It also talks of when peace came and the stories of how we got to that point, it's a way forward. When our kids are born and given the full truth of us as parents, they know we were not goodie two shoes all the time and we were not bad all the time either. It saves our children lots of "trial and error" time, to not make the same mistakes over again because that has already been tested. As we move in life we can figure out where the next bump on the road is and see if we jump over it, go around it, or do we get a shovel and level it out? We gather all the information to prepare our young and next generations how to see correctly and truthfully in the future. For Onkwehonwe, that is where all our data is—in the wampum itself.

Thomas R. Porter (Sakokwenionkwas, meaning "The One Who Wins") was the founder of the Mohawk Community of Kanatsiohareke (Ga na jo ha lay gay) in the Mohawk Valley near Fonda, New York (USA). He is a member of the Bear Clan of the Mohawk Nation at Akwesasne. Also known as the St. Regis Mohawk Reservation, Akwesasne straddles the New York State/Canadian border near Massena, New York (USA). Mr. Porter held the position of subchief for the Tehanakarine Chieftainship, one of nine chief titles of the Mohawk Nation, between 1971 and 1992. Mr. Porter was also the director of the Akwesasne Freedom School and a teacher at both the Akwesasne Freedom and the Kahnawake Survival Schools, where he taught Mohawk language, philosophy, history, and carpentry. Additionally, Mr. Porter worked as secretary for the Mohawk Nation Council of Chiefs for 8 years and as an interpreter for 11 years and counting. He organized the "White Roots of Peace," a traveling multimedia communications group designed to revitalize Native traditions and beliefs in North America. For 10 years, Mr. Porter was also the Native American consultant for the New York State Penitentiary System and Chaplain for all of the Native inmates in the New York State (USA) Penal System. Mr. Porter is a wealth of knowledge, and he makes ceremonial foods using the old traditional recipes and teaching it to the younger generation when requested. He is also an avid Rotinonshonni artist, creating beaded clan medallions and beaded tobacco/ prayer bags.

HRI Research, Inc This work was supported by HRI Research, Inc.

The manufacturer's authorised representative in the EU is Springer Nature Customer Service Centre GmbH, Europaplatz 3, 69115 Heidelberg, Germany. If you have any concerns regarding our products, please contact ProductSafety@springernature.com

Printed and bound by CPI Group (UK) Ltd, Croydon, CR0 4YY
07/07/2026
02160926-0002